T0270448

Beating Melanoma

A Johns Hopkins Press Health Book

Beating Melanoma

The Ultimate Patient Resource

Second Edition

Steven Q. Wang, MD

Johns Hopkins University Press

Baltimore

The names of the patients in this book have been changed to safeguard their privacy.

Johns Hopkins University Press
2715 North Charles Street
Baltimore, Maryland 21218
www.press.jhu.edu

Library of Congress Cataloging-in-Publication Data

Names: Wang, Steven Q., author.
Title: Beating melanoma : the ultimate patience resource / Steven Q. Wang, M.D.
Description: 2nd edition. | Baltimore : Johns Hopkins University Press, [2024] | Series: A Johns Hopkins Press health book | Includes bibliographical references and index.
Identifiers: LCCN 2023058728 | ISBN 9781421449876 (hardcover) | ISBN 9781421449487 (paperback) | ISBN 9781421449494 (ebook)
Subjects: LCSH: Melanoma—Popular works. | Melanoma—Treatment—Popular works. | BISAC: HEALTH & FITNESS / General | MEDICAL / Hematology
Classification: LCC RC280.M37 W35 2024 | DDC 616.99/477—dc23/eng/20240117
LC record available at https://lccn.loc.gov/2023058728

A catalog record for this book is available from the British Library.

Special discounts are available for bulk purchases of this book. For more information, please contact Special Sales at specialsales@press.jh.edu.

The facing page constitutes an extension of this copyright page.

To my mom and dad, I am eternally blessed by your love, wisdom, and guidance. With each passing year, I grow to appreciate more deeply all of your sacrifice, accomplishments, and character.

To my dearest Kevin, I am constantly amazed by your bravery and gentle kindness. I cannot wait to share with you all the magnificent wonders that this world has to offer.

To Kevin, Eric, and Elle, may you unlock your full potential, discover your true passion, and fulfill the bright destiny that awaits you.

To Dr. David Swanson, Dr. Stephen Dusza, Dr. Maryam Moinfar, Dr. Harold Rabinovitz, and Julie Bain for their critical reviews of the manuscript.

To my exceptional colleagues and friends who kindly volunteered their time and expertise to participate in the interviews for this book project. Thank you! Dr. David Polsky, Dr. David Swanson, Dr. Deborah Sarnoff, Dr. Douglas Grossman, Dr. Sancy Leachman, Dr. Thomas Wang, Dr. Trilokraj Tejasvi, Dr. David Fisher, Dr. Harold Rabinovitz, Dr. Justin Ko, Dr. Adam Friedman, Dr. Allan Halpern, Dr. April Salama, Dr. Chris Barker, Dr. Dan Coit, Dr. Henry Lim, Dr. Darrel Rigel, Dr. Laura Ferris, Dr. Paul Chapman, Dr. Peter Chen, Dr. Richard Carvajal, Kyleigh LiPira, and Dan Latore.

To the dedicated dermatology staff at Hoag Memorial Hospital Presbyterian in Irvine and Newport Beach, California, who are committed to delivering the best care to our patients every day.

To Suzanne I. Staszak-Silva, Alena Jones, and Robert Brown, my editors, for their professional excellence and for their many valuable suggestions.

Above all, to Maryam—the light of my life.

Contents

Preface

The incidence of melanoma has risen dramatically over the past 50 years; more and more people are developing melanoma. It is estimated that, in 2023, nearly 186,680 cases of melanoma will be diagnosed in the United States and that nearly 7,990 people in this country will die from it.

Melanoma can profoundly affect a person on many levels: physically, psychologically, emotionally, and economically. As a dermatologist and skin cancer specialist who worked at Memorial Sloan Kettering Cancer Center and is now working at Hoag Memorial Hospital Presbyterian, I have spent over 17 years of my career focused only on the prevention, diagnosis, and treatment of melanoma and other types of skin cancer. My work brings me into close contact with patients who share their stories with me. These stories are moving, inspirational, and, sometimes, sad. These interactions and experiences have given me a deep appreciation for and understanding of the difficulties and challenges that many patients face, especially in the beginning, when they are diagnosed with melanoma.

When first diagnosed, my patients react with a range of emotions, from surprise, denial, frustration, and confusion to fear and even despair. This is not the time to panic, however. Denial is not an option. You need to take action and take action fast. Certainly your physician will urge you to undergo treatment as soon as possible—and urgency is necessary—but some of my patients say that they feel themselves losing control as soon as the process starts.

There is no doubt that you will go through an intense period from the time of diagnosis to the time you complete treatment. I call this phase the "mad rush." Many patients find this to be a highly stressful time. They must quickly learn about the disease, find experts near their home, and decide on treatment options. During treatment, many people feel that the process is chaotic and that they have lost control. Navigating the mad rush phase can be challenging, even for many health care professionals. That's why I wrote the first part of this book, chapters 1 and 2.

Chapter 2 provides a step-by-step plan through the mad rush phase. It will help you become familiar with the vocabulary of melanoma, relevant medical background and basic treatment options, and information about survival outcomes, tailored to different individuals' conditions and the stage of their illness. Such knowledge can be extremely helpful when you are moving through the mad rush phase.

After successfully completing this phase, many people with melanoma feel a transient relief. At some point after treatment, however, most people who have had melanoma grapple with a fresh wave of questions and nagging concerns. They wonder if they will develop new melanoma or get other skin cancers. They wonder whether they will need more treatments. They worry about whether their children or their siblings will also get skin cancer.

With each passing year after treatment, most melanoma survivors gain a deeper understanding of their disease and become more comfortable and reassured. They enter what I call the "marathon" phase. Information in the second part of this book, chapters 3 and 4, addresses many of your lingering concerns and questions. These chapters will help you develop habits and practices that can prevent additional skin cancer.

I want to say a few words about cancer and attitudes toward cancer. In the United States and many other countries, the word "cancer" still carries frightful connotations. Many people consider cancer to be a death sentence. Luckily, this is far from the truth. Modern medicine has made enormous strides in the diagnosis and treatment of cancer. Progress in computer technology, noninvasive imaging, immunotherapy, targeted therapy, and other new discoveries have changed the medical management of cancers. In fact, I would even go so far as to state that many types of cancer have been transformed into chronic, rather than terminal, diseases, much like high blood pressure and diabetes.

While melanoma is the most dangerous type of skin cancer, most people who are diagnosed early have excellent prognosis and survival outcomes. Treatment for early melanoma is straightforward and not complicated. Because of heightened public awareness of the signs of skin cancer and improved diagnostic techniques, more people today are diagnosed at an early stage. If you are diagnosed with melanoma at an early or intermediate stage of the disease, it can be treated relatively easily. And treating cancer early usually means you will have an excellent chance for survival.

What Is New to the Second Edition of the Book?

The first edition of this book was published in 2011, and in the 13 years since then, significant changes have taken place in the realm of melanoma diagnosis and treatment.

First of all, the most noteworthy change is the emergence of immunotherapies and targeted therapies, which have revolutionized the treatment of advanced melanomas. These novel medications are nothing short of miracles, as they have substantially increased the survival rate of patients with metastatic melanoma from a few months to several years. Moreover, a considerable number of patients with advanced melanoma have been cured completely, which was not possible with any treatments available at the time the first edition was published. The second edition elucidates the mechanisms of action of these drugs and provides the latest clinical data on survival rates for different stages of melanoma.

Second, during the interim period, I have accumulated a wealth of knowledge and insights from treating thousands of patients with melanoma and non-melanoma skin cancers. This clinical and research experience has afforded me a deeper understanding of the challenges faced by my patients, an unwavering conviction that we can beat this disease, and a sense of humility over just how much we still do not know. I sincerely hope that all my experience can provide clarity, guidance, and hope for those who read this book.

Third, in preparing the second edition, I conducted interviews with 25 world-renowned experts in dermatology, surgical oncology, medical oncology, radiation oncology, genetics, dermatopathology, and nonprofits concerned with skin cancer. These experts practice at distinguished medical institutions across the nation, and most are highly published researchers and clinicians who have delivered numerous lectures in the United States and internationally on melanoma prevention, diagnosis, and treatment. Several of them have also served on expert panels for reputable organizations such as the American Joint Committee on Cancer and the National Comprehensive Cancer Network for melanoma. As a reader, you will have access to all of these interviews and be able to listen to the interviewees' candid and insightful discussions on a range of melanoma-related topics. Trust me, you will greatly benefit from the collective wisdom and experiences of these distinguished experts.

How to Read This Book

If you have just been diagnosed with melanoma and have not yet received any treatment, you are in the "mad rush" phase. I recommend that you first read chapter 1, which is a brief introduction to melanoma, and then read chapter 2, the step-by-step guide. Focus on understanding terminology and the tasks ahead.

Chapters 1 and 2 will help you work better with the team of physicians who will provide your treatment. You may want to read chapter 2 more than once, for better understanding. When you have completed your treatment or you have more time, read the rest of the book. Be sure to use the "Beating Melanoma Checklist" in chapter 5.

If you had melanoma years ago and were treated for it, you are in the "marathon" phase. I recommend that you read chapter 1 and then skip to chapters 3 ("The 'Marathon'

Phase: Surviving Melanoma") and 4 ("Networking: Finding and Sharing Information"). After you have read these chapters, you may find it helpful to read chapter 2 and complete some of the tasks described there, such as obtaining a copy of your old pathology report. Please also review the appendixes, which describe skin cancers other than melanoma.

Of course, you can read this book in the traditional fashion, from beginning to end. It is important, though, to read it a few times, because stressful situations impair our ability to absorb new information. To help you understand the medical terminology scattered through the book, you will find definitions of the terms in the book's glossary.

Finally, this book is accompanied by a set of video-recorded interviews available on BeatingMelanoma.com. As you read the chapters, you will come across prompts where I direct you to watch interviews I conducted with one or more of the melanoma experts whose names and affiliations are listed in the next section. These casual but comprehensive interviews offer insight into aspects of melanoma that may be hard to grasp fully in a written format. Therefore, I highly recommend that you watch these videos to enhance your understanding of melanoma.

Melanoma Experts

Dermatology

Laura Ferris, MD, PhD	Professor of Dermatology, University of Pittsburgh
David E. Fisher, MD, PhD	Edward Wigglesworth Professor and Chairman, Department of Dermatology, Harvard Medical School; Director, Melanoma Program, and Director, Cutaneous Biology Research Center, Massachusetts General Hospital
Adam Friedman, MD	Professor and Chair of Dermatology, Residency Program Director, Director of Translational Research, and Director of the Supportive Oncodermatology Program, Department of Dermatology, George Washington University School of Medicine and Health Sciences

Douglas Grossman, MD, PhD — Professor of Dermatology, Investigator, and Co-leader of the Melanoma Center, Huntsman Cancer Institute, University of Utah

Allan C. Halpern, MD, MSc — Chief, Dermatology Service, Department of Medicine, Memorial Sloan Kettering Cancer Center

Justin Ko, MD, MBA — Clinical Professor, Department of Dermatology, and Director and Chief of Medical Dermatology, Stanford Medicine

Sancy Leachman, MD, PhD — Professor and Chair, Department of Dermatology, and Director, Melanoma and Skin Cancer Program, Knight Cancer Institute, Oregon Health & Science University

Henry Lim, MD — Program Director, Dermatology Research, Program Director, Photomedicine Fellowship, and Ex-chair, Department of Dermatology, Henry Ford Health

David Polsky, MD, PhD — Professor of Dermatology and Pathology, Alfred W. Kopf, MD, Professor of Dermatologic Oncology, Director, Pigmented Lesion Section, and Vice Chairman for Research,

Ronald O. Perelman Department of Dermatology, Laura and Isaac Perlmutter Cancer Center, New York University Grossman School of Medicine, NYU Langone Health

Harold Rabinovitz, MD — Associate Clinical Professor of Dermatology, University of Miami School of Medicine; Professor of Dermatology, Medical College of Georgia

Darrell S. Rigel, MD — Clinical Professor of Dermatology, Mount Sinai Icahn School of Medicine

Deborah S. Sarnoff, MD — Clinical Professor, Department of Dermatology, New York University School of Medicine; Director, Dermatologic Surgery, Cosmetique Dermatology, Laser & Plastic Surgery, LLP; and Co-editor-in-chief, *Journal of Drugs in Dermatology*; and President, The Skin Cancer Foundation

David L. Swanson, MD — Professor of Dermatology, Residency Program Director, and Associate Director of Education, Mayo Clinic in Arizona

Trilokraj Tejasvi, MD — Associate Professor, Director, Cutaneous Lymphoma

Program, Director, Teledermatology Services, and Faculty Associate, Global REACH, Department of Dermatology, Michigan Medicine

Dermatopathology

Jerad M. Gardner, MD

Section Head of Bone and Soft Tissue, Pathology at Geisinger Medical Center

Medical Oncology

Richard D. Carvajal, MD

Deputy Physician in Chief and Director of Hematology and Medical Oncology, Northwell Health Cancer Institute; Roy J. and Tara Zuckerberg Professor in Medical Oncology, Donald and Barbara Zucker School of Medicine at Hofstra/ Northwell

Paul B. Chapman, MD

Chief Medical Research Officer, Meyer Cancer Center at Weill Cornell Medicine and NewYork-Presbyterian Hospital; Medical Oncologist and Attending Physician, Department of Medicine, Memorial

Sloan Kettering Cancer
Center; Professor of Medicine,
Weill Cornell Medical College

April K. S. Salama, MD   Associate Professor of Medicine, Division of Medical Oncology, and Director, Melanoma Program, Duke Cancer Institute

Surgical Oncology

Daniel G. Coit, MD, FACS   Attending Surgeon, Department of Surgery, Memorial Sloan Kettering Cancer Center; Professor of Surgery, Weill Cornell Medical College

Thomas N. Wang, MD, PhD   Director, Melanoma and Skin Cancer Program, Surgical Oncology, Hoag Family Cancer Institute, Hoag Memorial Hospital Presbyterian

Radiation Oncology

Christopher A. Barker, MD   Vice-Chair, Clinical Research, Department of Radiation Oncology, Memorial Sloan Kettering Cancer Center

Peter V. Chen, MD   Radiation Oncology, Hoag Family Cancer Institute, Hoag

Memorial Hospital
Presbyterian

Genetic Counseling

Jeanne Homer, Licensed
Certified Genetic Counselor

Hoag Family Cancer
Institute, Hoag Memorial
Hospital Presbyterian

Nonprofit Organization

Dan Latore

Executive Director, The Skin
Cancer Foundation

Kyleigh M. LiPira, MBA

CEO, Melanoma Research
Foundation

Beating Melanoma

1. Introduction

You Have Melanoma. Now What?

Stephanie was a 31-year-old woman with light blonde hair, deep blue eyes, and fair skin. She grew up in the city of Tinton Falls, a quaint and vibrant beach town in New Jersey. Growing up, she was a lifeguard and loved the outdoors. She lived near the ocean, where she had plenty of sun exposure and a few sunburns over the years. At the age of only 26, she had her first melanoma diagnosed and treated on her left leg.

This was Stephanie's third visit to our skin cancer clinic, where she was due for her quarterly skin exam to check that the melanoma on her left leg had not returned. Equally important, we needed to make sure she did not have any new melanomas or any other type of skin cancer.

Dressed in a hospital gown, she seemed at ease and smiled as I walked into the exam room. After learning about her promotion at work, the stress of balancing work and family life, and her daughter's latest mischievous deeds, I proceeded with the medical visit.

To start, I asked Stephanie a series of medical questions to assess her overall health. Then I started my skin exam and proceeded through my usual routine. Stephanie assured me that she was using sunscreen every day as I looked over all the moles on her arms and back with a dermatoscope. When I told her that I did not spot any concerning lesions on her upper body, she became a bit more relaxed, but I still sensed a guarded tension.

As I moved to examine her legs, I took a closer look and felt the 2-inch-long scar on her left leg—the lasting remnant of her melanoma surgery—to check for any recurrence of the melanoma. Next to that scar was a slightly atypical mole, measuring about 8 millimeters in size. As I studied the mole through the special lens of my dermatoscope, Stephanie became silent and still. That mole was benign, not worrisome. Sensing her anxiety, I assured her that everything looked good.

After finishing the skin exam, I again informed her that she was doing very well. The scar on her left leg was well healed. I did not see any moles or spots that were worrisome. As she listened to me, her eyes and left hand wandered to the scar on her left leg. I reminded her that it had been more than five years since her melanoma was diagnosed and treated. Now that she had passed that important five-year mark, her risk of the melanoma coming back had decreased significantly. More importantly, her risk of dying from this melanoma had dropped to an exceedingly low probability.

As we spoke, tears of joy and relief streamed down her cheek.

Stephanie's melanoma had been diagnosed in a fortuitous way. At the time she was working as a pharmaceutical representative, visiting doctors to educate them about the latest drugs from her company. One summer, a nurse at one of the offices pointed out a dark mole on her left leg and urged her to see a dermatologist. Heeding the warning, Stephanie made an appointment with a local dermatologist for three weeks later. The doctor removed the mole on the leg on that visit.

One week after the visit, the dermatologist shared the bad news: "Stephanie, the mole we removed from your leg is a melanoma. It is a type of skin cancer that needs to be treated quickly . . . We will refer you to Dr. Samson, a surgeon. He will excise it for you. This is his office number . . . We will also let him know . . ."

Stephanie was stunned by the news and did not recall anything else the doctor had said. When she hung up the phone, all she remembered was that melanoma is a dangerous type of skin cancer. Judging by the urgent tone in her dermatologist's voice, she knew the situation was serious. She made a note about the need to set up an appointment with the surgeon, but she was not sure what that visit would mean.

That night after dinner, she shared the news of the diagnosis with her husband. They had heard of melanoma but did not know much else about it. Soon, both Stephanie and her husband had a long list of questions, but it was too late to call her dermatologist. So they started googling on their phones. Jumping from one website to another, they tried to learn as much as possible about melanoma. They struggled with medical terms such as "Breslow thickness," "sentinel lymph node biopsy," "immunotherapy," and "melanoma-specific survival." The scariest moments were when they started reading blogs and social media posts detailing stories of young and healthy women whose lives had ended unexpectedly because of melanoma. They finally decided to stop the search after seeing some YouTube videos on skin surgery.

Stephanie recalled the harrowing experience of sitting beside her husband and sifting through those sites. The information was inconsistent. The medical terminology confused her. The statistics terrified her. To make matters worse, some of the reputable sites repeated similar warnings. All she could think about was the impending surgery. She wondered, "Is surgery enough? Do I need radiation? What about chemotherapy?" Before heading to bed, she stood over her baby daughter, who was sound asleep. She tucked the covers over her daughter's shoulder, kissed her forehead, and prayed silently.

Two weeks later, Stephanie met the surgeon, who explained the procedure to remove the melanoma, and learned about the risks associated with the surgery. Ten days later, she underwent the surgery in an ambulatory surgery center. Two weeks after that, she went back to the surgeon's office to have the sutures removed. These six weeks were insane. It seemed that her life was centered on going to the surgeon's office. Everything was a big blur.

Stephanie was lucky. Her melanoma was diagnosed at an early stage. She was cured by the surgery. There was no need for lymph node biopsy or other treatments. To this day, Stephanie was grateful for that nurse who had saved her life by warning her about the lesion.

Stephanie's experience is all too common. Many melanoma patients go through a similar phase of riding an emotional roller coaster. Upon hearing the diagnosis, many are shocked by the news. Next, waves of worry and fear set in. They are not only worried about themselves, but they also wonder what will become of their loved ones should they have a bad outcome.

Eventually, they shake off those dark feelings. Some simply accept the news and place all their faith and trust in their doctors. Many try to educate themselves, learning as much about this disease as possible. The journey of self-education is not easy. Although there are many educational resources available, the information is scattered and fragmented. Some sources are too superficial while others are too esoteric and hard to understand. Still others are outdated or simply inaccurate.

My own preference is that you should learn as much as possible about melanoma. The act of learning is empowering and can distract your mind from all the fears and worries. Knowledge is power. Soon you will meet different types of physicians who will examine you, talk with you, and work with you to come up with the best treatment plan. You will encounter unfamiliar medical terminology, treatment options, and statistics. You will have to make some serious decisions. And all of this will happen quickly. Being prepared for it will help you to make better-informed decisions.

There are other common themes during this journey. The period from the initial diagnosis to the final treatment is arduous. It is emotionally taxing and disruptive, as many patients have to prioritize their treatment and put other aspects of life on hold. It often seems as though all they are doing is visiting doctors. Moreover, they have to make important decisions about their treatment—and make them fast.

For all these reasons, I called this phase the "mad rush." Because you are reading this book, it is likely that you or someone you love is going through the mad rush phase. To help make this journey easier, you deserve to have a personal melanoma expert to act as an educator, navigator, and emotional supporter by your side. The next chapter is my attempt to offer such a companion to you.

In chapter 2, I outline a five-step plan to help you find needed information and make informed decisions during the mad rush. The five steps are these:

Step 1. Understand the Diagnostic Information in the Pathology Report

Step 2. Understand the Severity of Your Melanoma with the AJCC Staging System

Step 3. Understand Your Treatment Options

Step 4. Understand Survival Rate and Prognosis

Step 5. Find the Clinical Experts in Your Area

2. The "Mad Rush" Phase
Navigating with the Five-Step Plan

If this is your first melanoma, you may not feel prepared for what is coming your way. It is absolutely normal to feel shocked and overwhelmed. Your temperament, life experience, and support system will influence how you respond. It is also understandable that everyone will react differently and on a different schedule. My advice, though, is not wait too long with melanoma.

Summon up your courage and faith. Act quickly. You have to believe that you will not only survive but thrive. You have the potential to become stronger and more resilient and reassured when you emerge from the "mad rush" phase. So let us get started. Remember, in most cases, melanoma is highly curable, especially when it is diagnosed early and treated promptly.

Step 1. Understand the Diagnostic Information in the Pathology Report

Typically, up to this moment, you have received only *oral* confirmation of a melanoma diagnosis from your dermatologist. What you need now is the pathology report to document it. There is a lot of information in that *written* report. The additional information will help to (1) stage your disease (i.e., classify your melanoma according to how it is likely to behave), (2) decide on your treatment plan, and (3) predict your survival outcome.

Aside from these three important reasons, here two other practical reasons why you need to get the pathology report:

1. The report will make your upcoming doctor visits more efficient by preventing potentially dangerous delays.
2. The report will be essential for your long-term care.

In the coming weeks, you will likely meet with a few physicians from different specialties, possibly at different medical institutions. At each encounter, the physician will need to have access to the same basic information from the pathology report. The physicians cannot rely on your recollection; they need the written report for medical and legal reasons to plan treatment options. Without it, they cannot effectively devise a personalized treatment plan. If you do not have the pathology report in hand, the physician's office staff will have to track it down from the dermatologist who performed the initial skin biopsy. This could delay your care if tracking it down takes days.

After you complete the "mad rush" phase, you will need ongoing care, in what I consider the "marathon phase," which I discuss in chapter 3. The marathon phase may last decades and include follow-up visits with dermatologists and other physicians. During that time, you may relocate to another city, change physicians, or have other medical conditions that will change your life in unpredictable ways. As you meet with each new physician, that provider may wish to review the pathology report to learn more details about your melanoma. These new physicians may not trust your memory, and neither should you. It's human nature to forget crucial pieces of information contained in the pathology report.

Now comes the easy part: how to get a copy of the pathology report. Just ask the dermatologist or other physician who performed the initial biopsy. By law, the physician must give you a copy if you request it. Many medical offices and hospitals have electronic portals where you can directly access and download a copy of your pathology report. You should make a few hard copies for your records or save the electronic copy on your phone or computer.

Understanding the Report

At first glance, the report may be intimidating. *Do not* let all the medical language discourage you.

Find your pathology report now, if you have it, and follow along as I explain the sample report in figure 2.1a and b. Please note that different pathology labs use different formats; your report may look different. The crucial information may appear in different locations in your report, but the same elements should be there.

Basic Information

First, verify that (1) your name, (2) date of birth, and (3) the date when the biopsy was performed are accurate. It is necessary to confirm the accuracy of these three pieces of information because you want to be sure that this report is for you and not for someone else.

Next, make sure the correct anatomic location is listed. If the biopsy you had was on the leg, make sure the report states "leg" rather than some other part of the body. Also check that the side of the body listed (left versus right) is correct. As a dermatologic surgeon, I have occasionally seen mistakes about this in pathology reports, and it can cause a delay in treatment. If you see an error in the anatomic location, notify your physician to get it corrected. Simply call your doctor's office and say, "I noticed the pathology report states that the biopsy site is on my left leg. I think there is a clerical error. My biopsy scar is on my right leg."

The report should contain the name and contact information for the physician who performed the biopsy. There should also be the name and contact information for the pathologist or dermatopathologist who made the diagnosis.

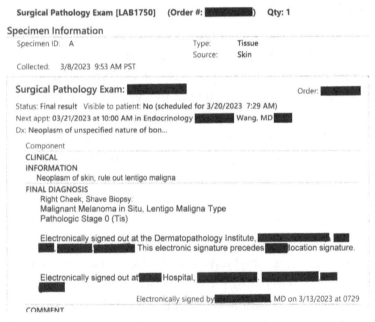

Figure 2.1a. Example of a pathology report showing a melanoma in situ.

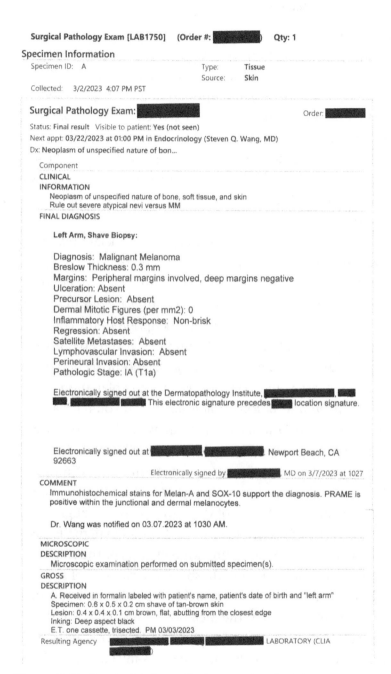

Surgical Pathology Exam [LAB1750]   (Order #: ███████)   Qty: 1

Specimen Information

Specimen ID: A		Type:	**Tissue**
		Source:	**Skin**

Collected: 3/2/2023 4:07 PM PST

Surgical Pathology Exam: ████████████   Order: ████████

Status: **Final result**   Visible to patient: **Yes (not seen)**
Next appt: 03/22/2023 at 01:00 PM in Endocrinology (Steven Q. Wang, MD)
Dx: Neoplasm of unspecified nature of bon...

Component
CLINICAL
INFORMATION
  Neoplasm of unspecified nature of bone, soft tissue, and skin
  Rule out severe atypical nevi versus MM
FINAL DIAGNOSIS

Left Arm, Shave Biopsy:

Diagnosis: Malignant Melanoma
Breslow Thickness: 0.3 mm
Margins: Peripheral margins involved, deep margins negative
Ulceration: Absent
Precursor Lesion: Absent
Dermal Mitotic Figures (per mm2): 0
Inflammatory Host Response: Non-brisk
Regression: Absent
Satellite Metastases: Absent
Lymphovascular Invasion: Absent
Perineural Invasion: Absent
Pathologic Stage: IA (T1a)

Electronically signed out at the Dermatopathology Institute, ████████████, ████
███, ████████████ ████ This electronic signature precedes ████ location signature.

Electronically signed out at ████████████ ████████████ Newport Beach, CA
92663
                                Electronically signed by ████████, MD on 3/7/2023 at 1027
COMMENT
  Immunohistochemical stains for Melan-A and SOX-10 support the diagnosis. PRAME is
  positive within the junctional and dermal melanocytes.

  Dr. Wang was notified on 03.07.2023 at 1030 AM.

MICROSCOPIC
DESCRIPTION
  Microscopic examination performed on submitted specimen(s).
GROSS
DESCRIPTION
  A. Received in formalin labeled with patient's name, patient's date of birth and "left arm".
  Specimen: 0.6 x 0.5 x 0.2 cm shave of tan-brown skin
  Lesion: 0.4 x 0.4 x 0.1 cm brown, flat, abutting from the closest edge
  Inking: Deep aspect black
  E.T. one cassette, trisected. PM 03/03/2023
Resulting Agency   ████████████ ████████████ LABORATORY (CLIA
                   ████████)

Figure 2.1b. Example of a pathology report showing an invasive melanoma.

Diagnosis and Description

Each report contains the same necessary elements: *diagnosis, macroscopic description,* and *microscopic description.* The macroscopic description provides details about the tissue specimen when it first arrived in the laboratory, before the tissue was processed in any way (i.e., before it was cut and stained). You do not need to understand the macroscopic description, so focus instead on the diagnosis and microscopic description. Below are 10 items of importance.

1. *Diagnosis.* Make sure the diagnosis of melanoma or other diagnosis is clearly stated. If you do not see a diagnosis, it usually means that the pathologist could not definitively assign a diagnosis to your case. In place of a diagnosis, the pathologist may offer a long description in the commentary section to explain the findings. If you do not see a clear diagnosis of melanoma in the diagnostic section of the report, ask your dermatologist for an explanation.

2. *Is it "in situ" or lentigo maligna only?* If you have a diagnosis of melanoma, the next question is whether the melanoma is in situ. This information will appear in the diagnosis section of the report. The term "in situ" means that the melanoma has not penetrated beyond the epidermis (the outermost layer of the skin). Lentigo maligna is a specific type of melanoma in situ. Lentigo maligna tends to occur on chronically sun-exposed areas of the skin in older individuals. Figure 2.1a shows an example of a pathology report with the diagnosis of melanoma in situ.

The depth to which the melanoma penetrates the skin's layers is very important. The thicker the melanoma—in other words, how deeply the lesion has invaded the skin—helps to predict how the melanoma will act. If you see the phrase "melanoma in situ" or "lentigo maligna," and there is no mention of "Breslow thickness" in the report, then you have a very early stage of melanoma. By definition, lentigo maligna and melanoma in situ have no depth. The treatment for melanoma in situ is straightforward. In most cases, all you need is a simple surgery to remove it with a standard margin. (Margin is a measurement of normal-appearing skin surrounding the lesion that a surgeon removes along with the lesion.) For melanoma in situ or lentigo maligna, the margin is usually 5 mm (millimeters) in size. You do not need any other aggressive treatment, and your chances for survival and cure are excellent.

If your melanoma is in situ or lentigo maligna *only*, then you can skip items 3 to 10 below, as the information there will not apply in your case. You can move ahead to Step 2: Understanding the Severity of Your Melanoma with the AJCC Staging System.

In general, if a melanoma is not an in situ lesion or a lentigo maligna, it is an invasive lesion. Invasive melanoma means that the tumor has penetrated the epidermis—that is, gone below the first layer of the skin. If the report states "invasive melanoma," then look next for the phrase "Breslow thickness."

3. *Breslow thickness is one of the critical pieces of information that (1) identifies the stage of the disease, (2) determines treatment options, and (3) helps predict survival rate.* Seeing the phrase "Breslow thickness" in the report means the melanoma is invasive and has penetrated the first layer of the skin. Breslow depth measures the depth of penetration of the tumor cells, starting from the top of the epidermis to the deepest melanoma cells in the skin tissue (figure 2.2). The unit of measurement is millimeters (mm).

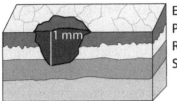

Epidermis
Papillary Dermis
Reticular Dermis
Subcutis (fat)

Figure 2.2. Breslow thickness measurement. The depth is measured in millimeters from the top of the epidermis to the deepest melanoma cells in the skin.

If you have trouble locating this information in your pathology report, look for a number followed by the abbreviation "mm" (for example, 0.5 mm, 1.2 mm, or 0.2 mm). Figure 2.1b shows an example of a pathology report with the diagnosis of invasive melanoma, and the Breslow thickness is 0.3 mm.

4. *Ulceration.* Ulceration indicates a loss of some of the skin that lies over the tumor. Patients who have melanoma with ulceration generally have a poorer survival outcome. Ulceration information is included in the report because it is needed to accurately categorize the stage of disease. If there is no ulceration, the report will say, "No ulceration present." If there is ulceration, the report will say, "Ulceration present."

5. *Mitotic rate.* Mitosis indicates that cells are undergoing division, splitting from one cell into two cells. Tumors grow by cell division, and the number of tumor cells undergoing mitosis reflects the activity of the tumor. Mitotic rate is an indicator of cell proliferation and is measured as the number of mitoses per millimeter squared. In the report, you will see this information presented as number/mm^2. In general, melanomas with a high mitotic rate are more aggressive and therefore more worrisome. According to the latest AJCC

(American Joint Committee on Cancer) guideline, mitotic rate is not a determining factor for staging the disease, but it remains a major determining factor that can influence survival outcome.

6. *Lymphovascular status.* The presence of melanoma cells in the lymphatic or blood vessels usually results in a worse outcome. It suggests that the tumor cells may have spread beyond the skin to other, distant parts of the body via either the lymphatic system or blood vessels. In most cases, though, there is no lymphovascular invasion. The pathology report would state, "Lymphovascular invasion is not identified."

7. *Regression* is defined by the presence of inflammation or scar tissue indicating that melanoma cells may have been destroyed by the immune system. Regression is either present or absent.

8. *Nerve involvement, or neurotropism,* refers to the presence of melanoma cells in the nerve fibers. "Neurotropism" is a term used by pathologist to describe the presence of melanoma in the nerve. In most cases, there is no nerve involvement.

9. *Margin status* comments on whether melanoma cells were observed in the periphery (i.e., edges) and depth of the biopsied specimen. In general, this information is not that important at the point of initial diagnosis, because in nearly all cases, the surgeon will perform an excision (a type of surgery) at a later time to remove the melanoma that includes an extra measure of the surrounding normal skin.

10. *Clark's level* is another way to describe the depth of melanoma invasion. This term is not generally used today and has largely been replaced by Breslow thickness. However, some pathologists may still report this information.

Please do not confuse Clark level with melanoma stage. The numeric designations for Clark level (I–V) mean something completely different from the stage of the disease (I–IV). For example, Clark level III does not mean stage III disease. The stages of disease are discussed in Step 2: Understand the Severity of Your Melanoma with the AJCC Staging System.

For more information on the pathology report and the terms described above, please watch my interview with **Dr. Jared Gardner**, an expert dermatopathologist. You can also get a visual tour of what melanomas look like under the microscope (https://www.beatingmelanoma.com/jerad-m-gardener).

1. Scan the code
2. Find the expert
3. Watch the interview

Pathology reports vary in the amount of detail they include. Most will contain the information described in items 1 through 9 above. For staging purposes, any pathology report should have Breslow thickness, ulceration status (present or absent), lymphovascular status, and mitotic rate. For in situ melanoma, the information in items 3 to 10 may not be included in the report.

Assess the Reliability of the Diagnosis

Before I discuss the reliability of a pathology report and the accuracy of a diagnosis, let me briefly describe how a pathology report is generated.

After a dermatologist biopsies a skin lesion, the skin specimen is dropped in a small bottle filled with formalin (a preservative) and sent to a lab where a technician cuts it into very thin slices of 4 to 20 micrometers (µm) in thickness, which is thinner than the width of an average human hair. The slices are placed on glass slides and stained with dyes (e.g., hematoxylin and eosin) that make the features of the tissue more visible and distinct. Occasionally, other stains such as MART-1, SOX-10, or PRAME are added to help differentiate a melanoma from a benign mole. I mention these special stains because they may show up on your pathology report.

The processed specimen on the glass slides is then sent to a medical specialist, either a pathologist or a dermatopathologist, who examines the tissue under a microscope. This pathologist considers the appearance of the tissue, focusing on the shape and structure (called "morphology") of the cells and tissue in the specimen. Based on these microscopic observations about the specimen, the pathologist reaches a diagnosis and records it in the pathology report. This report is then sent to the dermatologist who performed the biopsy.

Which Specialist Made the Diagnosis?

The terms "pathologist" and "dermatopathologist" both refer to physicians who examine tissue under a microscope, render a diagnosis, and generate pathology reports. What is the difference between them?

Pathologists are trained to examine tissue from all parts of the human body, such as the brain, muscle, colon, heart, and bone. By and large, most pathologists do not specialize in looking at skin tissue and may not examine it on a daily basis. In contrast, dermatopathologists are dermatologists or pathologists who have received additional training in examining skin specimens. In general, dermatopathologists are more knowledgeable when it comes to skin disease. The important point, though, is not whether a pathologist or a dermatopathologist reviewed the slides and made the diagnosis but rather whether they are experienced and knowledgeable when it comes to melanoma.

Why Does It Matter Which Pathologist?

A diagnosis should be made by an experienced and knowledgeable pathologist or dermatopathologist to avoid an error. Diagnosing melanoma can be challenging. There are a number of benign tumors that can mimic the appearance of melanomas. In addition, biology is not black or white. On the spectrum of benign to malignant lesions, there is often a large "gray" area where the clinical, pathological, and biological behaviors of lesions cannot be clearly defined. This can result in either over-diagnosis or under-diagnosis of melanoma.

The fact that melanoma diagnosis can vary between pathologists was illustrated in a clinical study conducted by a group of medical researchers in the Netherlands. The investigators submitted nearly 2,000 lesion samples for a second opinion to the expert dermatopathologists and pathologists of the Dutch Melanoma Working Group Pathology Panel. The experts changed the diagnoses in 27 percent of the cases—more than one in every four. Thus, it matters greatly that you get an accurate diagnosis from a specialist experienced in diagnosing skin cancer based on biopsied tissue.

Personally, I have seen quite a few cases where the initial diagnosis of melanoma was reversed or vice versa. I can still recall one of my young patients who wept tears of relief after learning that she did not have a deeply invasive melanoma. Instead, she had a Spitz nevus (a benign lesion with some features similar to melanoma). Her initial diagnosis was reversed after her slide was reviewed by a second, more experienced dermatopathologist. As a result, she did not need to undergo a large excision, sentinel lymph node biopsy, or other more aggressive treatment. (I explain sentinel lymph node biopsy in Step 3: Understand Your Treatment Options.) This second opinion averted an extensive surgery, potential additional treatments, and the lifelong label of melanoma survivor.

You want an expert who can accurately measure the Breslow thickness of the melanoma. In certain cases, measuring the deepest tumor cells in the skin tissue can be a challenge. As in many highly skilled tasks, experience and knowledge matter in taking this measurement. Overestimation of the Breslow thickness can lead to an unnecessarily aggressive surgery with a bigger surgical scar and longer recovery time. On the other hand, underestimation of the Breslow thickness can lead to inadequate and inappropriate treatment, which has the potential of allowing the melanoma to recur or to spread to other parts of the body.

How to Verify the Accuracy and Confidence of the Diagnosis

The easiest approach to verifying a diagnosis is to ask your dermatologist or the physician who performed the biopsy of the skin lesion. *Ask whether he or she trusts the diagnosis. Also ask if he or she has confidence in the pathologist or dermatopathologist who made the diagnosis.* As mentioned before, if you see a long description in the comment section rather than a clear diagnosis in the report, you may want to verify the accuracy and degree of certainty of the findings.

What to Do If You Are Not Satisfied with the Diagnosis

If the pathology report is unclear or is unsatisfactory to you in any way, you or your physician may wish to seek a second opinion. This is a common practice. A second opinion does not mean another skin biopsy. The same slides, taken from the original biopsy, can be sent to another pathologist or dermatopathologist for an independent review of the slides and a separate diagnosis. To request a second opinion, tell your physician, "Please have the slides reviewed by another dermatopathologist to confirm the diagnosis." These are the words that many dermatologists use when talking to each other about difficult cases.

If you don't feel comfortable using this direct language, here is another way to make the request: "Dr. [last name], I trust your judgment. Do you think it may be a good idea to ask another dermatopathologist or pathologist who is experienced in melanoma to review the slides and to confirm the diagnosis?" Remember that you want a board-certified and experienced dermatopathologist or pathologist to review your slides.

If you and your physician decide to have the slides reviewed by a second pathologist, it is important to move quickly. The process can take up to two weeks after initiating the consult for a second reading of the specimen. So, if you have doubts about the diagnosis, do not delay in discussing it with your physician.

When you receive the second diagnosis from your physician, proceed again with Step 1: obtain a copy of the pathology report and examine the information it contains. Now you will have two reports in hand. Compare the diagnoses and other findings in these two reports. Your dermatologist should explain the results to you in detail. In checking the second pathology report, here are few important steps:

- Again, confirm that the report is for you, not someone else.
- Check the *pathology accession number* in both reports. The accession numbers on both reports should be identical. This confirms that that the second dermatopathologist looked at the same specimen.
- Make sure that the report is for a sample from the correct anatomical site. For example, if you had three biopsies (e.g., right cheek, right arm, and left leg) but only the lesion on the left leg was in question, make sure the second report is for the left leg and not one of the other lesions. Such mistakes are rare, but they *can* happen.
- If the diagnosis is melanoma, is it invasive or in situ? If invasive, compare the measurement of Breslow thickness with that in the first report.

If the two pathology reports state the same conclusion, you will have more confidence in the accuracy and reliability of your diagnosis.

What to Do If the Reports Conflict

On rare occasions, two pathologists examining the same slides will have different findings and offer different diagnoses. If you obtain a second pathology report that differs from the first report, you can have a third dermatopathologist or pathologist review the slides. Ask your dermatologist for advice and guidance.

Step 2. Understand the Severity of Your Melanoma with the AJCC Staging System

Melanoma is a disease that presents with a wide range of severity. Fortunately, the majority of patients with early-stage disease have excellent prognosis. In contrast, patients with late-stage disease tend to have a worse prognosis. Accurately categorizing patients according to the severity of their disease can help to (1) predict survival, (2) personalize treatment options, (3) design and analyze clinical trials, (4) and plan for future follow-up.

The American Joint Committee on Cancer's staging system for melanoma is used to achieve all of these goals. The AJCC system has been revised a number of times. The latest edition, the eighth version, was implemented in the United States on January 1, 2018. The staging system was created by the Melanoma Expert Panel, which consisted of 37 physicians and statisticians. The latest version of the system was updated based on analysis of 46,000 patient records from 10 institutions in the United States, Europe, and Australia. The committee wanted the staging system to be practical and applicable to the needs of various medical specialties. The committee also wanted the staging criteria to reflect the biology of melanoma.

In the next section I explain the AJCC staging system for melanoma. Just a quick warning, though: the information is complex and can be difficult to comprehend. Do not get discouraged; just keep going, and it will all make sense in the end after I provide a few examples in the section "Putting It All Together" on page 33.

Understanding the staging system will give you a sense of the severity of your melanoma. More importantly, it can help to foster a more productive discussion when you meet with your physicians to decide on the best treatment options for you. *Please be aware, however, that the information below does not cover all the questions and nuances associated with melanoma staging. Ultimately, your doctors are the ones who have to stage your disease accurately and design the optimal treatment plan for you.*

Elements of the AJCC Staging System—TNM Status

The AJCC melanoma staging system consists of two systems: (1) clinical staging and (2) pathologic staging. Both systems are based on the TNM (tumor, nodes, metastasis) status of the melanoma. Clinical staging is conventionally used after the initial biopsy of the melanoma. Pathologic staging includes additional information from the surgical excision to remove the melanoma plus any pathologic information about regional lymph nodes after sentinel lymph node biopsy or complete lymph node dissection. For simplicity of discussion, I explain here only the pathologic staging system:

1. T stands for *primary tumor status* and includes
   a. Breslow thickness
   b. Presence or absence of ulceration

2. N stands for *regional and non-regional lymph node metastatic status* and includes:

   a. Regional lymph node, which is subdivided into

      i. Clinically occult nodal involvement—melanoma found only after sentinel lymph node biopsy (SLNB. See explanation in the next section.)

      ii. Clinically detected nodal involvement—that is, melanoma found on clinical exam (such as feeling the neck, armpits, or groin area) or radiologic imaging studies

   b. Non-regional lymph node, which is subdivided into

      i. Presence of in-transit metastases

      ii. Presence of satellite metastases

      iii. Presence of microsatellite metastases—that is, any microscopic focus of metastatic melanoma cells in the skin or subcutaneous tissue adjacent or deep to, but discontinuous from, the primary melanoma

3. M stands for *distant metastases*—that is, the tumor is found to have spread to other organs, such as the brain, liver, or lung. Imaging studies, such as a PET/CT scan or MRI, are used to find metastatic melanoma tumors in those distant organs.

A table of the TNM classification for melanoma (table 2.1) is available at BeatingMelanoma.com/Tables.

Clinically Occult versus Clinically Detected Lymph Node

For most patients, T status and M status are easily understood, but N status often requires more explanation. Specifically, the difference between clinically occult versus clinically detected lymph nodes can be confusing for patients.

To determine whether melanoma cells have spread from the primary site on your skin to the lymph nodes, your physician will exam your groin, armpits, and around the neck for any enlarged lymph nodes. Melanomas on the legs can travel through the lymphatic channels and spread into the lymph nodes in the groin area. Melanomas on the arms can spread to lymph nodes in the armpits. Melanomas on the trunk tend to spread to the armpits or groin nodes. Melanomas on the face, head, and neck can travel to the lymph nodes around the neck. It is important to note that not all melanomas start in the skin, and melanomas can arise from other non-skin sites such as the mucosal or uveal regions.

If your physician feels enlarged lymph nodes on clinical examination, additional procedures (e.g., core biopsy, fine needle biopsy, or excisional biopsy) are needed to sample and study the enlarged lymph node. If melanoma cells are confirmed in the enlarged lymph node, then the patient is said to have **clinically detected** lymph node involvement.

If, however, your physician does not find any palpable (i.e., detected by touch) lymph node or note any on imaging, that means you do not have a clinically detected lymph node. However, there is still a possibility that melanoma cells have spread to one of the regional lymph nodes and can only be detected after a surgical procedure called *sentinel lymph node biopsy*, or SLNB for short.

The presence of melanoma cells in a lymph node found after SLNB defines **clinically occult** nodal disease. Clinically occult nodal disease can only be detected by this surgical procedure. Clinically occult disease represents the majority of findings for patients who are initially diagnosed with regional lymph node metastasis.

In summary, clinically detected lymph node means that melanoma cells are present in a lymph node, as found by clinical exam or imaging studies. Clinically occult lymph node involvement, by contrast, means that melanoma cells were found in the sentinel lymph node only after a sentinel lymph node biopsy was performed.

What Is a Sentinel Lymph Node Biopsy?

The sentinel node is the first lymph node that melanoma cells reach when they spread away from the original site on the skin or elsewhere. To determine which is the sentinel lymph node that needs a biopsy, a surgeon injects a small amount of a radioactive substance, occasionally combined with a blue dye, at the site of the melanoma. The radioactive material and/or blue dye are then used to trace the flow of lymph fluid from the tumor to one of the lymph basins (in the neck, groin, or armpit, depending on the site of the tumor).

After making an incision in the lymph node region, the surgeon looks for lymph nodes blue in color or uses a radioactive probe to locate any "hot" (i.e., radioactive) lymph nodes. A hot node or a node that looks blue is regarded as the sentinel lymph node. That node is removed, processed in a lab, and then examined under a microscopic by a pathologist or dermatopathologist.

Lymph node status is one of the strongest prognostic indicators (predictive of survival). Many patients, especially young and healthy patients, with certain features of melanoma want to know their risks. Knowing offers peace of mind if they have no lymph node involvement.

As with any surgery, there are serious potential negative effects associated with this procedure. Overall, the risk of this procedure is relatively low, estimated to be 5–10 percent of cases. Most common complications include infections, poor wound healing, fluid accumulation at the surgical site (seroma), and lymphedema (swelling caused by a buildup of lymph). Some of these complications eventually resolve, but some can last indefinitely. Other less common risks include numbness, bleeding, and blood clots. For more details on the procedure, please watch my interviews with colleagues **Dr. Daniel Coit** (https://www.beatingmelanoma.com/daniel -g-coit) and **Dr. Thomas Wang** (https://www.beatingmelanoma .com/thomas-n-wang).

1. Scan the code
2. Find the expert
3. Watch the interview

You will need to have a discussion with your surgeon, oncologist, or dermatologist to determine if you need the SLNB procedure and to understand the relative risks and benefits associated with it.

Who Needs a Sentinel Lymph Node Biopsy?

It is important to know that **not every melanoma patient needs an SLNB.** Your physician may consider many factors before recommending that you have this surgery. In most cases, the decision to perform an SLNB is straight-forward. In other cases, though, the decision may be difficult, so you and your physician will need to discuss the pros and cons thoroughly.

Below are the recommendations from the 2022 National Comprehensive Cancer Network (NCCN) Guidelines for determining which patients should undergo SLNB. Most of the criteria come from information included in the pathology report for an initial biopsy.

1. SLNB is *NOT needed* for patients with melanoma in situ or lentigo maligna.
2. SLNB is *NOT recommended* for patients with melanoma measuring < 0.8 mm in Breslow thickness and without ulceration. This is because the probability of finding a positive SLNB for such patients (i.e., finding melanoma in the lymph node or having clinically occult lymph node) is < 5 percent. If there is significant uncertainty about the adequacy of microstaging, however, your physician may discuss your having an SLNB.
3. SLNB should be *considered* for patients with melanomas with the following T status:
   a. < 0.8 mm in Breslow thickness with ulceration
   b. 0.8–1.0 mm in Breslow thickness with or without ulceration

   This recommendation is based on the fact that patients in these categories have a 5–10 percent probability of having a positive SLNB. There are a number of adverse factors that may push your physician toward recommending SLNB, such as lymphovascular invasion or a mitotic index of > $2/mm^2$. Both lymphovascular invasion and mitotic index status are found in the pathology report.
4. SLNB should be *offered* to patients with melanomas having a Breslow thickness of > 1 mm regardless of

the ulceration status. In this case, the probability of having a positive SLNB is > 10 percent, and the risk increases as the Breslow thickness increases. However, if you are not physically or medically fit to act on the information from an SLNB, such as by going through adjuvant therapy, immunotherapy, or a complete lymph node dissection, then you and your physician may decide to forgo it.

The bottom line is that, with reference to the NCCN Guidelines, you and your physician(s) will decide on the best course of action for you.

AJCC Stages of Melanoma

I have taken a long detour to explain TNM status, the SLNB procedure, and the criteria for recommending an SLNB. This explanation is necessary for you to understand the staging process and treatment plans. Let us turn now to how physicians determine the stage of melanoma according to the latest AJCC staging system. Knowing the stage of melanoma will help to determine the optimal treatment course and prognosis. This is what your physician will do with every melanoma patient.

Below are the criteria for each stage of melanoma. As a reminder, I discuss here only the pathologic staging system, not the clinical staging system. As a reminder, T stands for tumor, N stands for nodal status, and M stands for distant metastasis.

Stage 0. A patient in this stage has an in situ melanoma (another name is lentigo maligna). This is a melanoma that has not penetrated beyond the epidermis (the first layer of the skin), and it can be treated easily. Patients with this stage of melanoma have excellent survival outcomes. In this stage, there is no evidence of lymph node involvement (N0) or distant organ involvement (M0).

Stage IA. A patient in this stage has melanoma with the following T status:

1. T1a: Breslow thickness < 0.8 mm with no ulceration
2. T1b: Breslow thickness < 0.8 mm with ulceration or Breslow thickness 0.8–1 mm with or without ulceration

There is no evidence of lymph node involvement (N0) or other distant organ involvement (M0). Example of stage IA: a melanoma of 0.5 mm Breslow thickness either with or without ulceration.

Stage IB. A patient in this stage has melanoma with the following T status:

1. T2a: Breslow thickness > 1.0–2.0 mm with no ulceration

In this stage, there is also no evidence of lymph node involvement (N0) or other distant organ involvement (M0). Example of stage IB: melanoma of 1.5 mm Breslow thickness without ulceration.

Stage IIA. A patient in this stage has melanoma with the following T status:

1. T2b: Breslow thickness > 1.0–2.0 mm with ulceration
2. T3a: Breslow thickness > 2.0–4.0 mm with no ulceration

In this stage, there is no evidence of lymph node involvement (N0) or other distant organ involvement (M0). Examples of stage IIA: (1) melanoma of 1.7 mm Breslow thickness with ulceration or (2) melanoma of 2.2 mm without ulceration.

Stage IIB. A patient in this stage has melanoma with the following T status:

1. T3b: Breslow thickness > 2.0–4.0 mm with ulceration
2. T4a: Breslow thickness > 4.0 mm and with no ulceration

In this stage, there is no evidence of lymph node involvement (N0) or other distant organ involvement (M0). Examples of stage IIB: (1) melanoma of 2.7 mm Breslow thickness with ulceration (2) or melanoma of 4.2 mm without ulceration.

Stage IIC. A patient in this stage has melanoma with the following T status:

1. T4b: Breslow thickness > 4.0 mm with ulceration

In this stage, there is no evidence of lymph node involvement (N0) or other distant organ involvement (M0). Example of stage IIC: melanoma of 4.4 mm Breslow thickness with ulceration.

Stage III. Melanoma in this stage displays regional lymph node (N) metastases, non-regional lymph node (N) metastases, or both. Stage III is separated into four subgroups, stages IIIA–IIID, based on tumor thickness, ulceration status, and the number and combinations of regional and/or non-regional lymph node metastases. In this stage, there is no evidence of other distant organ involvement (M0).

Again, as a reminder, regional lymph nodes include:

a. Clinically occult nodal involvement—confirmed ONLY after a sentinel lymph node biopsy

b. Clinically detected nodal involvement—found on clinical exam or radiologic imaging studies

Non-regional lymph nodes include:

a. Presence of in-transit metastases
b. Presence of satellite metastases
c. Presence of microsatellite metastases—that is, any microscopic focus of metastatic tumor cells in the skin or subcutaneous tissue adjacent or deep to, but separate from, the primary melanoma.

Example of stage IIIA: melanoma of 1.3 mm Breslow thickness without ulceration and one clinically occult lymph node (i.e., positive SLNB). Example of stage IIIB: melanoma of 1.4 mm Breslow thickness with ulceration and one clinically detected lymph node.

Stage IV. A patient with this stage has melanoma displaying distant metastasis to skin, soft tissue (e.g., muscle), or organs (e.g., lung, liver, or brain). The T status and the N status are not important. Only the M status (i.e., melanoma has spread to distant part of the body) matters. The M status is further classified into the following four groups:

M1a: spread to skin or soft tissue including muscle
M1b: spread to lung
M1c: spread to non-brain visceral sites, such as the liver
M1d: spread to the brain

Elevation of lactate dehydrogenase (LDH), a biological blood marker, is also used to subcategorize within each of the four groups. Example of stage IV: melanoma of 1.8 mm Breslow thickness with ulceration and metastatic disease in the lung.

A table briefly summarizing the melanoma pathologic staging system (table 2.2) is available at BeatingMelanoma .com/Tables.

Putting It All Together

To make sure that you have a good idea about how staging works, I present three clinical examples by way of illustration.

> **Scenario 1: Anthony** is a 39-year-old man who has a biopsy-proven melanoma on the left back. From the pathology report, I learn that the Breslow thickness is 0.5 mm and the tumor is not ulcerated. Clinical examination of both armpits does not reveal any palpable lymph nodes.
>
> In this case, Anthony has T1a (i.e., Breslow thickness < 0.8 mm) and stage IA disease. A SLNB procedure is not recommended in this case because the Breslow thickness is < 0.8 mm. **He has stage IA disease.**
>
> **Scenario 2: Samantha** is a 47-year-old woman who has a biopsy-proven melanoma on the right leg. From the pathology report, I learn that the Breslow thickness is 1.2 mm and the tumor is not ulcerated. Clinical examination of the right groin does not find any palpable lymph nodes. Based on the pathology report, Samantha has T2a (i.e., Breslow thickness > 1 to 2 mm and no ulceration) and stage IB disease.
>
> Because the Breslow thickness of the melanoma is greater than 1 mm, however, she is a good candidate for SLNB to make sure she has no clinically occult

lymph node involvement. She undergoes the SLNB procedure. The final AJCC stage depends on the SLNB finding. *If her SLNB is negative, then her stage of disease remains IB; if her SLNB is positive, she will be upgraded to stage III.*

Scenario 3: Jeff is a 67-year-old man who has a biopsy-proven melanoma on the scalp. From the pathology report, I learn that the Breslow thickness is 1.8 mm with ulceration. Clinical exam around the neck does not find any palpable lymph nodes. He subsequently undergoes SLNB, which is positive (i.e., detection of a clinically occult lymph node). Jeff has stage IIIB disease because he has T2b (> 1–2mm thick with ulceration) and N1a (one clinically occult lymph node).

Although Jeff does not complain of any symptoms that suggest spread of the disease to other distant organs, his physician decides to proceed with baseline imaging studies, such as PET scan, CT scan, and/or MRI. The final staging depends on the results of the imaging studies. *If the imaging studies show that no other organs are involved, then his stage remains IIIB; if, however, imaging shows that melanoma has spread to other organs, such as the lung or the liver, Jeff will be upgraded to stage IV disease.*

I hope these three clinical examples help you in tying together all the information about staging. Again, please rely on your treating physicians to determine your stage. Based on the stage of the melanoma, your physicians will decide on the optimal course of treatment.

Step 3. Understand Your Treatment Options

Optimal treatment options are determined by the stage of the melanoma. For early-stage melanoma, excision with a margin is all that is needed. For advanced melanoma, however, systemic treatments, such as immunotherapy, targeted therapy, or radiation, are required.

The following paragraphs outline the treatments for different stages of melanoma, taken from the NCCN Guidelines published in 2022. *The treatment outline is intended as an informational guide only. It does NOT cover all the nuances associated with melanoma treatment. It CANNOT replace the recommendation from your doctor who knows your specific melanoma and can design an optimal treatment plan. In addition, your doctor knows about your overall health, other medical issues, and social conditions.* Do not be surprised if two patients with the same stage of disease receive different recommendations for treatment. *Listen to those clinical experts who are treating you.* Lastly, modern medicine progresses at an extraordinarily fast pace. Other cutting-edge treatments may be available at the time you are reading this book.

As a reminder, there are two different staging systems. For simplicity and consistency in discussion, I refer here to the pathologic staging system.

Stage 0

Patients in stage 0 have melanoma in situ or lentigo maligna. In stage 0, melanoma cells have not penetrated beyond the epidermis (the first layer of the skin). The treatment plan is relatively straightforward: remove the melanoma with a standard surgical margin of 0.5–1 cm (figure 2.3 and table 2.3). "Standard surgical margin" refers to the amount of normal surrounding skin tissue that needs to be removed. Routine imaging (e.g., X-ray or CT scan) or lab tests are not recommended.

As mentioned earlier, lentigo maligna is a type of melanoma in situ commonly found on sun-damaged skin, such as on the face. Like all melanoma in situ, patients with lentigo maligna have a superb prognosis. However, the challenge when treating lentigo maligna is that it is often difficult to tell where the cancer stops and normal tissue starts. As a result, the standard margin of 0.5 to 1 cm may not be adequate.

There are instances where surgery is not a suitable option because the lentigo maligna is too large to be completely removed. Also, in some cases, after the initial surgery, the pathology report may show that the tumor has not been completely removed. In those cases, a topical drug, imiquimod (Aldara), is often prescribed. The drug works on cell

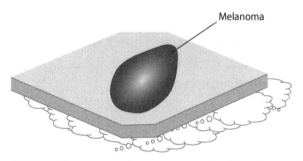

Melanoma

Figure 2.3. An illustration showing a surgical excision of a melanoma with the appropriate surgical margins. Melanoma (*black*) is located in the center of the ellipse. A margin of normal surrounding tissue (*gray*) outlines the appropriate surgical margins.

Table 2.3. Surgical Margins for Wide Excision of Melanoma Based on Breslow Thickness

Breslow thickness of tumor	Recommended peripheral surgical margin
In situ	0.5–1 cm
<1.0 mm	1 cm
>1.0–2.0 mm	1–2 cm
>2.0 mm	2 cm

surface molecules associated with immune response, called the Toll-like receptors, and activates immune cells to destroy the remaining cancer cells. Although this drug is not approved by the FDA to treat melanoma, studies have shown high rates of melanoma clearance and low recurrence rates. For additional detail on the treatment of lentigo maligna with imiquimod, please watch my interview with **Dr. Allan Halpern** (https://www.beatingmelanoma.com /allan-c-halpern). In addition to imiquimod, radiation is another treatment option. For details on the use of radiation treatment, please watch my interviews with **Dr. Chris Barker** (https://www.beatingmelanoma.com/christopher-a -barker) and **Dr. Peter Chen** (https://www.beatingmelanoma .com/peter-v-chen).

1. Scan the code
2. Find the expert
3. Watch the interview

Stage IA

Stage IA includes two groups of patients. Those with T1a and those with T1b disease.

1. T1a disease has a Breslow thickness < 0.8 mm and no ulceration. For this group, treatment involves an

excision of the melanoma along with a standard surgical margin of 1 cm. Since the Breslow thickness is < 1mm, SLNB is not recommended, nor are routine imaging (e.g., X-ray or CT scan) or lab tests. No other treatment modalities, such as immunotherapy or targeted therapy, are needed.

2. T1b disease has a Breslow thickness < 0.8 mm with ulceration or a Breslow thickness of 0.8–1 mm with no ulceration. For this group, treatment involves an excision of the primary melanoma along with a standard surgical margin of 1 cm of normal surrounding tissue. SLNB is discussed and considered but not routinely offered. Routine imaging (e.g., X-ray or CT scan) or lab tests are not recommended. No other treatment modalities, such as immunotherapy or targeted therapy are needed.

In the following story, Gloria, one of my melanoma patients, details her surgical experience from a first-person perspective.

> **My melanoma was found** by my dermatologist during an annual skin exam. Right then he biopsied the worrisome lesion, which was on my right arm. One week later, he called me with the diagnosis of melanoma. I was very worried. He explained the biopsy results and said that the lesion needed to be removed, and soon. I was glad when he told me that the melanoma was relatively thin. It had a Breslow thickness of 0.2 mm. I did not really understand what that meant at the time. I do remember my dermatologist urging me not to go online and do too

much research. He warned me that potential misinformation on the web might scare me.

On the day of surgery, I was rather nervous. I arrived in his office 30 minutes prior to my scheduled appointment. His office staff asked me to fill out a questionnaire. Soon, a nurse brought me into a procedure room. The room was about 10 by 12 feet, clean and organized. It was not like those operating rooms you see on television shows or what I had imagined. Next, the nurse asked me a series of questions about my health, past medical history, allergies, and current medications. She was kind and gentle. Before leaving the room, the nurse gave me a gown to change into.

It was not long before my dermatologist walked into the room. He was wearing blue hospital scrubs instead of his usual white coat. He shook my hand and asked how I was feeling. Then he explained the diagnosis again and described the procedure he would be doing. He said that the surgery was fairly straightforward, yet there were potential risks, including pain, infection, bleeding, scarring, swelling, numbness, and the possibility of recurrence of the melanoma. His explanation was clear, but it also made me feel more anxious. When he asked if I had any questions, I shook my head and signed a consent form that allowed him to do the surgery.

I lay back in a very comfortable exam chair. The nurse positioned the chair in a fully reclined position and offered me a pillow for my head. Next, the doctor marked the site on my right arm and cleaned the area with alcohol. The smell and cold sensation made me a little anxious. He told me that he would give me a shot to numb the area. I felt only a tiny sting when he gave me the shot. I did not feel any pain after that. My doctor was constantly talking to me and letting me know what he was doing, and that helped me not to worry as much. Soon, my arm felt like it was getting swollen. The doctor assured me that feeling was a normal sensation.

Next, I heard him opening the tray of surgical instruments, but I did not want to see them. A few sterile blue towels were placed on my right arm, and he cleaned the area again with some different fluid this time. The nurse asked me what music I would like to hear. I thought to myself that I didn't care; anything would be fine. Seeing my hesitation, she suggested something soothing, and I agreed. I felt my doctor and his assistant touching my arm as the nurse started the music. Next, the doctor looked at me and said, "Gloria, we are doing well. I already removed the tumor."

Naturally I was surprised that it was gone already. I then felt some tugging in my right arm and sensed that the arm was getting tighter. I did not feel any pain, however. My doctor reassured me that everything was going well. Five to 10 minutes later, he told me that the procedure was over. I was relieved.

My doctor gave me some instructions on how to care for the wound, showed me the surgical site where he had removed the lesion, and shook my hand before leaving the room. The nurse then cleaned the area around the wound and put a bandage over it. She went over the wound care instructions again and gave me a written instruction sheet. She said that I could take some Tylenol if I had pain but not to take Advil (ibuprofen), because ibuprofen can increase the risk of bleeding. I got out of the comfortable chair, changed back into my clothes, and thanked everyone in the office.

Overall, my experience was great. That night I experienced some minor pain, so I took two Tylenol and applied some ice to the area. It didn't hurt much after that. Two weeks later, I went back to the dermatologist's office. He took out the sutures and told me that all the cancer had been removed and that the margins were free of any melanoma. I felt like a heavy weight had been lifted off my shoulders.

Stage IB

Patients with stage IB disease shows T2a disease, defined as Breslow thickness > 1.0–2.0 mm and with no ulceration. The treatment for stage IB consists of a standard excision of the tumor along with a standard surgical margin of 1 to 2 cm. SLNB is discussed and offered to the patient because the Breslow thickness of the primary melanoma is > 1 mm. Routine imaging (e.g., X-ray or CT scan) or lab tests are not recommended. No other treatment modalities, such as immunotherapy or targeted therapy, are needed.

Stage IIA

Patients with stage IIA disease consists of two groups. Those who have T2b disease or T3a disease.

1. Patients with T2b disease have Breslow thickness 1.0–2.0 mm with ulceration. For this group, treatment involves an excision of the tumor along with a

standard surgical margin of 1–2 cm. SLNB is discussed and offered. Routine imaging (e.g., X-ray or CT scan) or lab tests are not recommended. No other treatment modalities, such as immunotherapy or targeted therapy, are needed.

2. Patients with T3a disease have Breslow thickness 2.0–4.0 mm with no ulceration. For this group, treatment involves an excision of the tumor along with a standard surgical margin of > 2 cm. SLNB is discussed and offered. Routine imaging (e.g., X-ray or CT scan) or lab tests are not recommended. No other treatment modalities, such as immunotherapy or targeted therapy, are needed.

Stage IIB

Patients with stage IIB disease consist of two groups. Those who have T3b disease or T4a disease.

1. Patients with T3b disease have Breslow thickness 2.0–4.0 mm with ulceration. For this group, treatment involves an excision of the tumor along with a standard surgical margin of 1–2 cm. SLNB is discussed and offered. Routine imaging (e.g., X-ray or CT scan) or lab tests are not recommended by the NCCN Guidelines, but some physicians may order baseline imaging studies.

2. Patients with T4a disease have Breslow thickness > 4.0 mm and no ulceration. For this group, treatment involves an excision of the tumor along with a standard surgical margin of > 2 cm. SLNB is discussed and offered. Routine imaging (e.g., X-ray or CT scan) or

lab tests are not recommended according the NCCN Guidelines, but some physicians may order baseline imaging studies.

For patients with stage IIB, your physician may also discuss additional (adjuvant) treatment with immunotherapy (see page 46). The goal of adjuvant therapy is to prevent melanoma from coming back after surgery. Locoregional radiation therapy has been used as well, but it has very limited role.

Stage IIC

Patients with stage IIC disease have T4b disease with Breslow thickness > 4.0 mm and ulceration. For this group, treatment involves an excision of the tumor along with a standard surgical margin of 2 cm. SLNB is discussed and offered. Routine imaging (e.g., X-ray or CT scan) or lab tests are not recommended according the NCCN Guidelines, but some physicians may order baseline imaging studies. Like the management for stage IIB, your physicians may discuss adjuvant immunotherapy (see page 46). Locoregional radiation therapy has been used, but it has very limited role.

Stage III

Patients with stage III disease have involvement of the regional lymph nodes. Stage III disease is further categorized into stages IIIA, IIIB, IIIC and IIID. The criteria for the different classifications are quite complex and depend on the number of lymph nodes involved and the T classification of the original tumor.

For patients with stage IIIA, imaging studies (e.g., CT, CT/PET, or MRI) should be considered for further baseline staging and to address any signs and symptoms reported by patients. For patients with stages IIIB/C/D, imaging studies (e.g., CT, CT/PET, or MRI) should be offered for baseline staging and to address any signs and symptoms reported by patients. For all stage III patients, testing for a *BRAF* genetic mutation of the tumor is performed. (For more on the *BRAF* mutation, see page 54.)

The primary treatment for stage III melanoma involves an excision of the primary tumor with a standard surgical margin of 1–2 cm. For melanoma with Breslow thickness between 1 and 2 mm, the standard surgical margin is 1 cm. For melanomas with Breslow thickness > 2 mm, the standard surgical margin is 2 cm.

With respect to treating the lymph nodes, there is an option of using ultrasound to monitor the lymph nodes for recurrence or, alternatively, a complete lymph node dissection to remove the rest of lymph nodes in the region. Historically, all patients with positive SLNB have been advised to receive a complete lymph node dissection, or CLND. However, several studies and clinical trials have changed current management decisions regarding CLND. These studies showed that CLND did not improve overall survival or melanoma-specific survival when compared with patients who were followed with clinical observation alone. As a result, a large percentage of surgical oncologists today do not elect to recommend CLND.

When compared to SLNB, CLND has significantly higher complication rates, ranging from 20 to 60 percent. These complications include poor wound healing, infection, bleeding under the skin, neuropathy (nerve injury), and lymphedema (swelling caused by a backup of lymph). Both neuropathy and lymphedema can be permanent. In some of the studies, the risk of lymphedema ranged from 20 to 50 percent for the patients who underwent the procedure. Risk factors and complication rates are correlated with increased age and obesity. For a more detailed discussion of SLNB and CLND, please see my interviews with surgical oncologist colleagues **Dr. Daniel Coit** (https://www.beatingmelanoma.com/daniel-g-coit) and **Dr. Thomas Wang** (https:// www.beatingmelanoma.com /thomas-n-wang).

1. Scan the code
2. Find the expert
3. Watch the interview

Your physician may discuss the options of adjuvant treatment, which is defined as treatment after the primary surgery with the goal of preventing melanoma from coming back to the local site. According to the NCCN Guidelines, adjuvant treatments include immunotherapy with either nivolumab (Opdivo) or pembrolizumab (Keytruda) or a combination of targeted therapy with dabrafeninb-trametinib for patients that have a tumor mutation called *BRAF* V600. It is important to mention that clinical observation is also an option according to the NCCN Guidelines. (I discuss immunotherapy and targeted therapy in more detail later in the chapter.)

As I have repeatedly stated, treatment decisions need to be individually tailored for a patient depending on the therapeutic goals and a patient's ability to tolerate these treatments. That is why it is important to consult your physicians, especially a medical oncologist, to decide which option is ideally suited for your melanoma.

Stage IV

Stage IV is disease that has spread beyond the regional lymph nodes to other parts of the body.

The initial workup includes imaging studies, such as CT, CT/PET, or MRI, which are needed to establish a baseline full staging of the disease and to address any signs and symptoms reported by patients. A test for *BRAF* mutation is performed on the tumor. Lastly, a lactate dehydrogenase blood test is performed.

Although a medical oncologist typically takes over the treatment plan at this point, patients with advanced stages of disease may first be presented at a multidiscipline tumor board meeting, where physicians from different specialties gather to review, discuss, and coordinate a care plan. In all cases, the care plan needs to be individually tailored for the patient depending on the therapeutic goals and the patient's ability to tolerate the treatments. In addition, the time may come to stop or switch therapies, depending on the progression of the disease and response to the treatments.

Next, I review four types of non-surgical therapies— immunotherapy, targeted therapy, chemotherapy, and radiation—that are used to treat advanced stages of melanomas. In general, immunotherapy and targeted therapy are used as the first and second line of treatment, respectively.

Immunotherapy

The immune system relies on coordinated actions from different types of immune cells (e.g., T cells and B cells) to seek and destroy bacteria, viruses, and even cancer cells. Immunity is a highly complex system that must work in

concert when an "enemy" such as an infection is identified, but the immune system must also know when to turn
itself off. Thus self-regulation is critical. Without it, normal tissues and organs will be damaged.

Cancer cells exploit the self-regulatory function of the
immune system and have developed a range of mechanisms to evade, thwart, or even hijack the body's immune
system, allowing cancer cells to further mutate and grow
unchecked. One such evasive action is sending a cellular
signal to the body's immune cells instructing them to
disengage and not to attack the cancer cells.

Immunotherapy is a medical breakthrough that prevents
immune cells from turning themselves off prematurely,
thereby maintaining an active, always-on mode to attack
the cancer cells. To take driving a car as an analogy, immunotherapy disengages the brakes of the car, allowing the
immune system to keep "driving" to identify and destroy
the cancer cells.

Immunotherapy drugs are super weapons against
advanced stages of melanoma, and they are also effective
in treating many other types of cancers. In fact, immunotherapy has been dubbed the fourth pillar of cancer
treatments, with the other pillar modalities being surgery,
radiation, and chemotherapy.

There is a rapidly growing number of immunotherapy
drugs for treating melanomas. The first two classes of drugs
block cytotoxic T lymphocyte antigen–4 (CTLA-4) or programmed cell death protein 1 (PD-1). CTLA-4 and PD-1 are
both receptors on T cells that normally limit or stop the
immune response. By blocking these two receptors with
drugs, the immune cells (T cells) are continuously activated.
Recently, two new classes of drugs have been approved by

the Food and Drug Administration (FDA). These drugs target the programmed death ligand 1 (PD-L1) protein on tumor cells and immune cells and the lymphocyte-activation gene 3 (LAG3) protein on immune cells.

Anti-PD-1 Drugs

Pembrolizumab (Keytruda) Pembrolizumab (Keytruda) from Merck is the first PD-1 antibody drug approved by the FDA to treat melanoma. Melanoma cells escape the immune system by attaching to the PD-1 receptors on T cells. Specifically, the PD-L1 and PD-L2 protein "ligands" (i.e., two molecules) on melanoma cell surfaces bind to the PD-1 receptors on the T cells like keys into locks. This binding action renders the T cells inactive and unable to detect and destroy the melanoma cells.

Keytruda binds to the PD-1 receptors on the T cells. Once that happens, the melanoma cells can no longer bind to the T cells. Now the T cells are continuously activated and remain effective in destroying the melanoma cells. Keytruda was first approved by the FDA in 2014 as a first-line treatment for advanced melanoma, specifically defined as stage III melanoma not able to be completely removed by surgery, and stage IV, or metastatic melanoma. The drug was then approved as adjuvant treatment for stage III melanoma in 2019 and for stages IIB and IIC melanoma in 2021. Again, the goal of adjuvant treatment is to prevent the melanoma from coming back after surgery.

Typically, the drug is given every three or every six weeks, delivered via infusion, whereby the drug is delivered into the bloodstream through an intravenous line. Each infusion is performed at an outpatient or ambulatory clinic, such as an infusion center, where a dedicated nursing staff can monitor the progress of patients. A typical infusion treatment lasts about 30 minutes.

Nivolumab (Opdivo) Opdivo is another anti-PD-1 drug from Bristol Myers Squibb, and it has the same mechanism of action as that of Keytruda. Opdivo binds to the PD-1 receptors on T cells, thereby preventing T cells from binding to the PD-L1 and PD-L2 ligands on melanoma cells.

Opdivo was first approved by the FDA in 2014 for previously treated metastatic melanoma. In 2016, the drug was approved for unresectable (i.e., not recommended for surgical removal) or metastatic melanoma regardless of *BRAF* status, either alone or in combination with ipilimumab (Yervoy). In 2017, it was approved for adjuvant treatment after surgery for patients with completely resected melanoma.

Like Keytruda, the drug is given as an intravenous infusion, usually every two or every four weeks, and each treatment usually lasts about 30 minutes.

Anti-CTLA-4 Drugs

Ipilimumab (Yervoy) Ipilimumab (Yervoy) from Bristol Myers Squibb is an antibody that binds to the CTLA-4 protein, a receptor on T cells. CTLA-4 is used by the immune system to temper its response to potential targets. CTLA-4 is on T cells and binds to the CD80/CD86 receptors on cells (called antigen-presenting cells, or APC) that are designed to inform the immune system of foreign or unusual antigens. When this happens, T cells activation is inhibited. To return to our car analogy, the brake is applied and immune system is stopped. When Yervoy binds to CTLA-4, however, it disables the brake. Now the T cells remain activated to seek and destroy melanoma cells.

Yervoy was first approved by the FDA to treat metastatic and unresectable melanoma in 2011. It was then approved as adjuvant treatment for melanoma after surgery in 2015. The drug is given as an intravenous infusion, usually every two to four weeks depending on the indication. Each infusion treatment usually lasts about 30 minutes.

Compared with Opdivo or Keytruda, Yervoy has much greater toxicity and less efficacy in extending overall survival. For these reasons, most oncologists prefer either Opdivo or Keytruda as the first line of treatment for unresectable or metastatic melanoma.

Nivolumab (Opdivo) + Ipilimuab (Yervoy) Combo The combination of these two immunotherapy drugs, nivolumab and ipilimuab, was first approved by the FDA to treat metastatic and unresectable melanoma in 2016 regardless of *BRAF* status.

In addition to these three immunotherapy drugs that work on the CTLA-4 and PD-1 proteins, there are two newer drugs that block the proteins PD-L1 and LAG-3 and deserve mentioning.

Anti-PD-L1 Inhibitor Drug

Atezolizumab (Tecentriq) targets the programmed death ligand 1 (PD-L1) protein on tumor cells and immune cells. The binding of PD-L1 on tumor cells with PD-1 on T cells causes the deactivation of the T cells. Blocking this binding reaction helps to reactivate and boost the immune response against melanoma cells.

Tecentriq is made by Genetech and received its approval from the FDA in 2020. This drug is given along with cobimetinib (Cotellic) and vemurafenib (Zelboraf) for patients with metastatic melanoma that have the *BRAF* mutation. (See page 54 on the mechanisms of Cotellic and Zelboraf.) Tecentriq is given as an intravenous infusion every three weeks.

LAG-3 Inhibitor Drug

LAG-3 is the abbreviation for the protein from lymphocyte activation gene 3. This is another protein on certain immune cells that inhibits or checks the immune system.

In 2022, the FDA approved the combination of relatlimab (LAG-3 inhibitor) and nivolumab (PD-1 inhibitor) for treating patients with metastatic melanoma or unresectable melanoma. This combination of two drugs, called Opdualag, is made by Bristol Myers Squibb. It is given as an intravenous infusion, typically once every four weeks.

For more details on why a medical oncologist would choose a single agent (e.g., Keytruda alone) versus dual agents (e.g., Opdivo and Yervoy in combination), please watch my interviews with colleagues **Dr. Paul Chapman** (https://www.beatingmelanoma.com/paul-chapman), **Dr. April Salama** (https://www.beatingmelanoma.com /april-k-s-salama), and **Dr. Richard Carvajal** (https://www .beatingmelanoma.com/richard -carvajal), medical oncologists who specialize in melanoma treatment.

1. Scan the code
2. Find the expert
3. Watch the interview

Talimogene Laherparepvec (T-VEC or Imlygic)

Before ending this discussion of immunotherapy options, there is one more drug that leverages the body's immune system to treat advanced melanoma. T-VEC or Imlygic is made by Amgen and was approved by the FDA in 2015 to treat stages IIIB/C and IV melanomas that cannot be completely resected with surgery. The drug can shrink melanoma tumors in the skin and lymph node but does not appear to improve overall survival.

T-VEC is made from a modified cancer-killing human herpes simplex virus 1 and can be injected directly into the melanoma in the skin, under the skin, or in the lymph nodes. After local injection, the virus replicates within the melanoma cells, rupturing and killing the tumor cells. In addition to causing melanoma cell death, T-VEC can also boost the body's immune response. When the melanoma cells are killed, melanoma antigens (proteins from tumor cells) are released into the circulatory system and potentially can attract and activate immune cells to attack the remaining melanoma tumor.

Unlike the other immunotherapy drugs mentioned above, T-VEC is delivered through a series of local injections. After the first injection, the second dose is given three weeks later, and all subsequent doses are given every two weeks.

Side Effects of Immunotherapy

As mentioned at the top of the section, immunotherapy drugs work by activating the body's immune system. One major category of their side effects is the high likelihood of immune cells attacking normal tissues and organs in any area of the body—an autoimmune reaction. These immune-related toxicities can be severe and even life-threatening. These immune reactions may be associated with any of the immunotherapy drugs: anti-CTLA-4, anti-PD-1, anti-PD-L1, or LAG-3 inhibitor.

Side effects on the skin are most common in the form of an itchy rash or blisters on the skin, even in the mouth, nose, eyes, or genital area. Impact on the respiratory system (e.g., lungs) can cause cough, shortness of breath, or chest pain. Attack on the gastrointestinal system can lead to diarrhea, liver damage, abdominal pain, or bloody stool. Immune reaction in the endocrine systems may affect the thyroid, pituitary, or other hormone glands, which can cause a significant disruption to the body's hormonal balance.

For these reasons, patients undergoing immunotherapy need to be closely monitored by their physicians. On some occasions, immunotherapies may be temporarily or permanently stopped because of the severity of these toxicities. It is imperative that you tell doctors and nurses in the clinic or infusion center should you have symptoms such as trouble breathing, chills, itchy rash, blisters, cough, or diarrhea. Of all the side effects, pneumonitis (inflammation of the lung) and colitis (inflammation of the intestine) are very concerning. If you are taking immunotherapy and start to have loose stools (a symptom of colitis) or cough or shortness of breath (symptoms of pneumonitis), you should tell your physician immediately. Before starting these immunotherapy medications, your medical oncologist should review the potential side effects associated with these drugs.

Lastly, because of all these potential immune-related side effects, your physician needs to determine if you are a good candidate before starting you on this class of drugs. Your physician may ask if you already have an autoimmune disease, such as lupus, Crohn's disease, or ulcerative colitis. The last two are autoimmune diseases that affect the intestinal tissue. They may also ask if you ever had an organ transplant or bone marrow (stem cell) transplant or neurologic conditions such as myasthenia gravis or Guillain-Barré syndrome. Additionally, physicians will want to know if a female patient is pregnant.

For detailed discussion on the different types of immunotherapies, please see my interviews with medical oncologists **Dr. Paul Chapman** (https://www.beatingmelanoma.com/paul-chapman), **Dr. April Salama** (https://www.beatingmelanoma.com/april-k-s-salama), and **Dr. Richard Carvajal** (https://www.beatingmelanoma.com/richard-carvajal), in which they share their clinical experience.

1. Scan the code
2. Find the expert
3. Watch the interview

Targeted Therapy

Nearly half of all melanomas have a specific mutation in a gene called *BRAF*. Melanomas with this mutation are labeled as having the *BRAF* V600 mutation (where 600 refers to the location of the mutation, specifically amino acid number 600 on the protein). It may be hard to imagine that a single tiny change in a gene sequence could cause the development and spread of melanoma.

Targeted therapy, as the name suggests, uses drugs that target and destroy melanoma cells with this specific *BRAF* V600 mutation. The two classes of drugs that target this genetic pathway are BRAF inhibitors and MEK inhibitors.

The BRAF inhibitors are vemurafenib (Zelboraf), dabrafenib (Tafinlar), and encorafenib (Braftovi); they work by directly attacking the BRAF protein, thereby shrinking or slowing the progression of melanoma cells. These drugs come in the forms of pills or capsules, and the dosage is either once or twice a day. It is important to note that this class of drugs is given only to patients with melanomas that have the *BRAF* mutation. Hence, prior to prescribing the medication, the genetic profile of the melanoma is analyzed to make sure it has this mutation.

Some of the common side effects of BRAF inhibitors include itchy skin rash, development of non-melanoma skin cancer, fever, fatigue, or hair loss. Also, patients can experience increased sensitivity to the sun, leading to sunburn.

The BRAF inhibitors are approved to treat metastatic melanoma or unresectable melanoma. In clinical practice, the current standard is not to use these medications alone but rather in combination with MEK inhibitors. When BRAF inhibitors are given alone, they tend to work initially, but they quickly lose their effectiveness due to drug resistance. Progression of disease usually occurs within the first six months of starting a BRAF inhibitor. However, when BRAF inhibitors are combined with MEK inhibitors, studies have shown higher efficacy rates and fewer side effects.

The MEK inhibitor drugs are trametinib (Mekinist), cobimetinib (Cotellic), and binimetinib (Mektovi). They work by blocking MEK proteins and stopping the growth of melanoma cells. MEK inhibitors are nearly always given in combination with BRAF inhibitors. Here are the following combinations of BRAF and MEK inhibitors approved by the FDA:

1. dabrafenib + trametinib
2. vemurafenib + cobimetinib
3. encorafenib + binimetinib

For a detailed discussion on targeted therapy, please watch my interview with **Dr. Paul Chapman** (https://www .beatingmelanoma.com/paul-chapman), who conducted the clinical trial that led to the approval of the first BRAF targeted therapy.

1. Scan the code
2. Find the expert
3. Watch the interview

Chemotherapy

Prior to the era of immunotherapy and targeted therapy, chemotherapy drugs such as dacarbazine, temozolomide, paclitaxel, albumin-bound paclitaxel, carboplatin/paclitaxel, and cisplatin/vinblastine/dacarbazine were the only choices for patients with metastatic melanoma. Unfortunately, the efficacy of these chemotherapy drugs is rather poor. In current clinical practice, these chemo drugs are given only when immunotherapy or targeted therapy fails to control the spread of melanoma. Even then, many medical oncologists wish to explore clinical trials for other kinds of treatment.

Radiation

As mentioned before, surgery is often considered to be the first line of treatment for early-stage melanoma. Immunotherapy and targeted therapies are deployed as the first-line treatment for advanced stages of melanoma. In some situations, radiation therapy has an important role in melanoma care. Radiation is used in a number of clinical settings.

First, radiation is used as a definitive therapy to treat lentigo maligna, a type of melanoma in situ that is commonly present in elderly patients with extensive sun damage. This type of melanoma is usually superficial, large in size, and commonly found on the face. In some clinical situations, surgery is not a reasonable option because either the patients are too frail or the lesions are too large. In those settings, radiation can be used as a therapy with an intention to eradicate the disease completely.

Second, radiation is used as an adjuvant treatment after surgical removal of "desmoplastic" melanomas, an unusual subtype of melanoma typically found in the head and neck region, where adequate surgical margins may not always be possible. For example, a desmoplastic melanoma with a Breslow thickness of 3 mm may require removal of 2 cm of normal tissue all the way around the lesion. This wide margin may not be possible or desirable because it would encroach on cosmetically sensitive structures, such as eyelids, lips, or ears. In addition, desmoplastic melanoma has a high tendency to invade the surrounding nerve fibers, leading to a higher rate of local recurrence. For these reasons, radiation is often used as an adjuvant treatment, after the initial surgery, to prevent local recurrence of the melanoma.

Third, in patients with positive lymph nodes, radiation has been used in an adjuvant setting to treat the entire "nodal basin," which is defined as a group of lymph nodes that receives and filters lymph in a certain area of the body. The nodal basins include the head and neck region, armpit, and groin. Radiation to the head and neck and the armpit regions appears to have better efficacy in preventing recurrence of melanomas than it does to the groin. Also, radiation to these areas has been shown to have fewer side effects such as lymphedema. In contrast, there is significant morbidity associated with radiation to the groin nodal basin.

Lastly, radiation has been used with a palliative purpose to treat distant metastasis of melanoma. In this situation, the goal is not to achieve complete cure or prevent disease from recurring; rather the goal is to reduce pain and discomfort. Radiation has been used to treat bone, brain, and deeper tissue metastasis.

Radiation treatment is carried out under the direction of radiation oncologists. Working with a team of physicists, radiation oncologists plan the total radiation dose, number of treatments (called fractions), and modalities to deliver the treatment. A complete course of radiation treatment is often divided into sessions spanning weeks or months. One of the immediate and common side effects is inflammation of the irradiated area. The inflammation can look like severe sunburn, and the irradiated skin can break down, resulting in painful erosions or ulceration. Moisturizers and antibiotic lotions may be used to soothe and heal the area. Long-term side effects of radiation include darkening of skin color, scarring, and a bound-down appearance to skin. Perhaps the most troubling side effect is lymphedema, defined as the swelling of arms or legs from a backup of lymph. Massage and compression stockings can help to minimize the discomfort.

For more detailed discussion of the application of radiation in treating melanoma, please watch my interviews with **Dr. Chris Barker** (https://www.beatingmelanoma.com/christopher-a-barker) and **Dr. Peter Chen** (https://www.beatingmelanoma.com/peter-v-chen), who are radiation oncologists.

1. Scan the code
2. Find the expert
3. Watch the interview

In summary, I have reviewed the treatment options for patients with advanced stages of melanoma. The use of immunotherapy and targeted therapy has greatly improved the overall survival of melanoma patients, and these have become the first- and second-line treatment options. In nearly all cases, your medical oncologist will coordinate your care and discuss with you the risks and benefits of these systemic treatments. A face-to-face consultation is necessary for you to understand the treatment plans. You may be given a great deal of information at these consultations, so I recommend that you bring someone with you. A family member or friend can listen and take notes; afterward the two of you can compare your understandings of the information conveyed in the consultation. Getting a second or third opinion with other specialists in different medical centers can also be a good idea, but these additional consultations should proceed with a sense of urgency. You should not delay treatment.

Clinical Trials

Before I move on to Step 4: Understand Survival Rate and Prognosis, I want to quickly mention the role of clinical trials in the treatment of melanomas. Immunotherapy and targeted therapy are real game changers in the fight to treat patients with advanced stages of melanoma, but not every patient responds to these treatments. If the disease progresses and does not respond to treatment, one option to consider is looking for novel treatments being tested in clinical trials under way around the country. For more detailed information on clinical trial options, please watch my interviews with **Dr. Richard Carvajal** (https://www.beatingmelanoma.com/richard-carvajal)

and **Dr. April Salama** (https://www.beatingmelanoma.com /april-k-s-salama), who are medical oncologists. In addition, I want to share a website where you can search for various trials enrolling patients with different diseases: https:// clinicaltrials.gov/.

 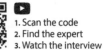

1. Scan the code
2. Find the expert
3. Watch the interview

Step 4. Understand Survival Rate and Prognosis

Prognosis means the probable outcome of a disease. This prediction can be measured in terms of cure rate, remission rate, recurrence rate, or survival rate. Although all of these measurements are valuable to researchers and clinicians when monitoring the progress of treatments, I focus here on overall melanoma-specific survival rate.

Our estimates for the survival rates of patients with different stages of melanoma come from the eighth edition of AJCC melanoma data, which were published in 2018, over half a decade ago. As I mention below, much has improved since then. A table presenting 5- and 10-year survival data from the AJCC (table 2.4) is available at BeatingMelanoma.com/Tables.

Patients with stage 0 melanoma (i.e., melanoma in situ or lentigo maligna) have excellent prognosis. There is virtually zero risk for metastatic spread. Although the eighth edition of the AJCC system does not specifically list the overall survival rate for patients with stage 0 melanoma, the 5-year survival is almost 100 percent.

Patients with stages IA and IB disease also have excellent cure rates. For stage IA, the 5-year and 10-year melanoma-specific survival probabilities are 99 percent and 98 percent, respectively. For stage IB, the 5-year and

10-year melanoma-specific survival probabilities are 97 percent and 94 percent.

Stage II melanoma has three separate subgroups. For stage IIA, the 5-year and 10-year melanoma-specific survival probabilities are 94 percent and 88 percent, respectively. For stage IIB, the 5-year and 10-year melanoma-specific survival probabilities are 87 percent and 82 percent. For stage IIC, the 5-year and 10-year melanoma-specific survival probabilities are 82 percent and 75 percent.

Stage III has four separate subgroups. For stage IIIA, the 5-year and 10-year melanoma-specific survival probabilities are 93 percent and 88 percent, respectively. For stage IIIB, the 5-year and 10-year melanoma-specific survival probabilities are 83 percent and 77 percent. For stage IIIC, the 5-year and 10-year melanoma-specific survival probabilities are 69 percent and 60 percent. For stage IIID, the 5-year and 10-year melanoma-specific survival probabilities are 32 percent and 24 percent.

For stage IV disease, the 5-year survival rate from the 2018 AJCC data was about 22 percent.

The survival rates for stage IV and late stage III disease can be disheartening. It is important to remember that these survival rates are based on the historical data and represent the best estimate available. This does *not* mean that all patients in a particular group will have the same outcome. There will always be exceptions in any statistical model. I have taken care of patients with very advanced stages of disease, and they have defied the statistical prediction and are still doing well decades after their initial diagnosis and treatment.

It is also important to remember that treatment options for advanced stages of melanoma are improving continuously. The survival rates given above are from the eighth edition of the AJCC data published in 2018. At the time I am writing this second edition in 2023, improved therapy protocols and newer drugs have already increased the overall survival rates for patients with advanced disease. There is good clinical evidence showing an improvement in survival rate for patients with late-stage melanoma reported in the five years since the 2018 data. Findings from leading academic centers have shown that the survival rate for advanced stages of melanoma have increased to 45 percent. For example, the Checkmate 067 clinical trial, using the combination of ipilimuab and nivolumab, found that patients achieved an overall survival of 49 percent for a period of seven and a half years.

Before I move on to Step 5, I want to emphasize that melanomas are not all the same. There is no doubt that melanoma is a very dangerous type of skin cancer when it is detected in later stages. Patients with early stages of the disease (e.g., stages 0 and I), however, have excellent cure rates. Early detection followed by prompt treatment saves lives and ensures the best clinical outcome with lowest morbidities. That is why it is a good idea to have a skin check done at least annually. In addition, if you are concerned about any suspicious skin lesions, do not wait. Call your dermatologist or primary care physician to have them checked out.

Step 5. Find the Clinical Experts in Your Area

Thus far I have discussed how to review the key information on a pathology report (Step 1). You have gained some idea of how to determine the stage or severity of your melanoma (Step 2). You learned, too, about various treatment options (Step 3) and the prognosis (Step 4) associated with each stage of the disease.

I have assumed up to this moment that you have only had an initial biopsy for diagnostic purposes and that you have not yet had definitive treatment for removal or treatment of the melanoma. As you embark on the treatment phase, finding clinical experts in your geographic area will be very important. As mentioned in Step 3, melanoma treatment options vary depending on many factors. These include Breslow thickness, mitosis rate, ulceration, anatomic location, your age and health, and stage of the disease.

The physician or team of physicians who take on your care will play a crucial role in the success of your outcome. Their expertise, judgment, and knowledge matters! Inadequate or ineffective treatment can potentially lead to recurrence or metastasis of the disease, which can be fatal. In contrast, overly aggressive treatment can lead to unnecessary physical and psychological trauma.

These points are illustrated by the following two stories. Stacy is my patient. Helen's story was related to me by an oncologist who runs clinical trials for patients with advanced stages of melanoma.

Stacy's and Helen's Stories

Stacy was a 32-year-old female and a melanoma survivor. Her melanoma (Breslow thickness 0.4 mm) was located on her left knee; it had been diagnosed and treated more than a year before I met her. Her treatment course was long and arduous, lasting nearly

a full year. After the initial biopsy, she soon underwent surgery to remove the tumor with standard
margins of normal tissue removed around the lesion.

Her recovery was complicated by poor wound healing. The scar spread open and took a month and a half
to heal. In addition, she had a sentinel lymph node
biopsy on her left groin. After the surgery, the surgeon
referred her for a chest CT scan. The CT scan showed a
few questionable spots in one of her lungs. Stacy
informed her doctor that she was a smoker, and her
doctor recommended that she have a total-body PET
scan to further examine those spots and check for
other irregularities. The PET scan showed that her
lung was normal, but it indicated that there was a
suspicious spot on her right ankle. She then proceeded
with an MRI and a bone scan to look for the "hot"
spot on her right ankle. Neither of these imaging
studies was definitive. To finalize the workup, she had
a bone biopsy on the right ankle, and the finding was
benign (normal). This ordeal took nine months in
which she went from one doctor to the next and had
one test after another.

After the diagnosis and treatment of her melanoma,
Stacy was told to have regular follow-ups with her
local dermatologist. She had many moles. On each
visit, her dermatologist found some moles that were
worrisome and removed one to three of them. All of
these subsequent biopsies were benign; the moles were
determined not to be melanomas. By the time I met
Stacy, she had at least 15 small scars variously located
on her body. Afraid of being "skinned alive," she came

to our dermatology clinic for a second opinion about continuing her follow-up.

Helen was a woman in her early thirties who lived in the United Kingdom. Her melanoma was diagnosed at a very late stage. She wanted to come to the United States to find a cure. Because of Helen's poor health, her doctors in the United Kingdom advised her not to make the transatlantic journey. Ignoring her doctors' warnings, she came to a specialty cancer institute in the United States. The repeated clinical workups, involving blood tests and a PET scan, confirmed that her melanoma had spread to her lung and liver.

Helen was immediately started on a cocktail of systemic drugs that targeted the melanoma cells, boosted her body's immune system, and slowed the growth of new blood vessels that would feed the tumors. Within three months, Helen's disease had melted away. Her follow-up PET scan showed clearance of the prior "hot" nodules in the liver and lungs. Her success story was nothing short of a miracle. The combination of treatments fought off the tumors.

Both women's stories are remarkable, and there is a stark contrast in their care. Stacy was subjected to overaggressive treatments. She had a very early disease. Her melanoma was only 0.4 mm in Breslow thickness, so she did not need a sentinel lymph node biopsy. No subsequent imaging studies were needed according to the current management guideline for melanoma. These additional studies led to an unnecessary bone biopsy and an invasive procedure that left Stacy with recurring pain in her ankle. It was extremely unlikely that an early melanoma on the left knee would jump and spread to the right ankle.

Moreover, imagine the fear, the sleepless nights, and the anxiety that she and her husband endured that year. Her dermatologist, in an effort to detect new melanomas, started to biopsy many benign moles and left her with many unnecessary scars on her body.

In contrast, Helen had seemingly terminal disease before being rescued by a team of specialists in melanoma care. Defying her own doctors' advice in England, she sought out the most expert care and became free of disease.

The point of sharing these two stories is neither to vilify nor to glorify any of the doctors involved. The simple message is this: *a qualified and expert team of physicians can ensure the highest chance for the best outcome.* Or, stated differently, when treated by inexperienced physicians, patients with any stage of melanoma may have worse outcomes. In Stacy's case, what should have been a straightforward treatment for an early melanoma turned into a year of continual tests, complications, and some unnecessary procedures. In Helen's case, a young woman with an advanced stage of disease found hope after her original doctors had nearly given up on her.

How to Find Experts near Your Home

There is no one way to find experts. Here are five suggestions.

First, specialists working in medical or cancer centers tend to have more experience in dealing with intermediate and advanced stages of melanoma. Most physicians in these types of institutions also have better ancillary support in treating people with melanoma. Often, the care provided in these institutions is orchestrated by a team of specialists, including dermatologists, medical oncologists, surgical oncologists, radiologists, radiation oncologists, dermatopathologists, and plastic surgeons, as well as nurses, psychologists, and social workers. Furthermore, some of these specialists have a strong clinical and research focus trained specifically on melanoma. They may have dedicated decades of their medical career to taking care of melanoma patients.

This is not to say that physicians who work outside major hospitals or cancer centers are not able to treat melanoma patients. In fact, many melanoma survivors are treated and cured by physicians who do not belong to these centers. Some of these physicians may even have spent years working in academic institutions or cancer centers before leaving them to pursue private practice or to work in other medical settings. Since melanoma is not a common disease, however, many community physicians, competent though they may be, have seen only a few cases over the course of their careers, especially late-stage melanoma. Physicians working at academic centers tend to see more cases, more complex cases, and have the facilities available to deal with many situations that arise.

Second, find experts by searching scientific publications listed in PubMed (https://pubmed.ncbi.nlm.nih.gov/) or in Google Scholar. Both sites are excellent resources for looking up the latest clinical and basic science research. Simply search with keywords, such as "melanoma treatment," "melanoma trials," or "melanoma diagnosis." You will see a long list of published articles. Now, look at the list of authors for these publications, especially the senior author, who is usually listed as the first or last author. Many of these authors are keenly interested in the diagnosis and treatment of melanomas, and many are experts recognized by their peers. Next, google their names to find their hospital affiliations and contact information.

Third, ask your dermatologist where you can receive the best treatment. For early-stage disease, many dermatologists will just excise the melanomas themselves. However, some may refer you to other specialists, such as a dermatologic surgeon, oncologic surgeon, or oncologists (cancer doctors) for definitive treatment.

You may like and trust your dermatologist, but how do you know if other specialists unfamiliar to you are qualified to diagnose and treat you? The quickest way to begin assessing the capability of those other physicians is to ask your dermatologist about them. Here are some helpful questions: How good is this surgeon or oncologist? How long have you worked with him or her? Better yet, ask, "Would you refer your own mother to see this specialist?" The last question is a litmus test. It is a good sign if the dermatologist looks you straight in the eye and tells you, "Yes, I would." In general, good physicians work with good physicians. Long periods of collaboration among different specialists reflect a sense of trust and approval for each other's work. No good physician will continue to refer his or her own patients to an unqualified physician.

Fourth, ask around. If you have friends or family members who had melanomas, call them. Ask about their experience. Get the name and contact information of their doctors. Word of mouth is often helpful.

Finally, if you have melanoma, ideally you will see a physician who is predominantly focused on treating melanoma and other types of skin cancer. Review the physician's biography to learn about his or her credentials, experience, and clinical interest. You can learn a great deal by visiting their websites. Focus on the overall appearance and content of the site. You can make some educated guesses about whether a particular doctor is suitable for you. For instance, if the site lists information only for cosmetic services, such as Botox and laser treatment, with no mention of skin cancer treatment, then this dermatologist is probably not the ideal person to care for your melanoma.

Independent third-party websites have been created to rank and review doctors. In my opinion, some of these sites do not provide objective assessments. In many cases, the posted comments remark mostly on a physician's bedside manner. These sites may be biased, since comments tend to come from patients who were either extremely pleased or extremely displeased with the doctor.

For more ideas on how to find an expert, please watch my interview with **Dr. Deborah Sarnoff** (https://www.beating melanoma.com/deborah-s-sarnoff).

1. Scan the code
2. Find the expert
3. Watch the interview

What to Do If You Cannot Find Experts near Your Home

If you live in an area where there are no melanoma experts, you may wish to seek care or a consultation in another city, depending on the stage of the melanoma. If you are able to travel, you can seek a consultation at an out-of-town institution, even if you don't live nearby. Experts there can make recommendations for a treatment plan, and then your local doctors can perform the treatment recommended by these experts. Many institutions now offer telemedicine with virtual visits.

Before closing this chapter on the five steps for navigating the "mad rush" phase of melanoma, I want to share a few more thoughts.

My first set of comments is for patients with early stages of melanoma. I understand the diagnosis can be highly unsettling, but please focus on the positive aspects. Remember that melanoma should not be viewed as a single disease. Different stages of disease require different treatments and have different survival outcomes. If you have early-stage disease, you need only a simple skin surgery to remove the melanoma. You do not need immunotherapy, targeted therapy, radiation, or chemotherapy. You should recover well and quickly. I often tell my patients to limit their online research because it tends to create unnecessary stress.

My next set of comments is directed to patients with an advanced stage of melanoma. The survival data for patients with melanoma at stage III or IV can be alarming and cause anxiety, but it is very important to remember that these statistics are only estimates, and, frankly, they do not reflect the current survival data. You are not a standardized number; you are a unique individual.

The statistical data help physicians choose optimal treatment options and estimate survival outcomes. Just in the past decade, the survival data for advanced melanomas have improved dramatically with the advent of immunotherapies and targeted therapies. Over this period, I have personally followed countless patients who beat their melanomas and achieved total cure. They defied statistics, fought their disease, and experienced remission or were even cured.

Modern medicine does not stand still. The pace of innovation is only accelerating. With each passing year, medical researchers have discovered additional novel strategies to treat melanoma. We have tweaked treatment plans to achieve better cure rates, while limiting potential side effects. I sincerely believe that the overall survival statistics will only improve in the coming years. I am not alone in this belief. This sentiment is shared by all of the melanoma experts I interviewed for this second edition, and many think we are at an inflection point where better treatments are around the corner.

Lastly, I believe that mental fortitude and personal mindset play an important role in clinical outcomes. Although we physicians design and deliver the treatments, what the patients bring mentally and emotionally to the therapeutic process makes a big difference. Nearly all of my patients who beat the odds found reasons to hope, to fight, and to live. So, whatever you do, remember to keep your spirits up. It is understandable that you will be tired and get scared at some points in the treatment process. Just do not let these fears hold you back for long. Remember to enlist family, friends, or a support group to give you the strength and hope to go forward.

3. The "Marathon" Phase
Surviving Melanoma

The "mad rush" phase of dealing with melanoma is a high-pressure, fast-paced period when most patients feel as though they are shuttling from doctor to doctor for workups and treatment. Many patients experience a sense of chaos and loss of control. The five-step plan in chapter 2 aimed to provide the necessary vocabulary and knowledge to help you navigate your way through this intense phase.

After successfully passing through the mad rush phase, many patients initially feel a sense of relief. Nearly all patients and their family members, however, have lingering concerns and new questions: Do I need any additional treatment? Is the melanoma really gone? Will it come back? How will I know if it comes back? How can I protect myself from developing additional melanomas in the future? Are my children or other family members at risk for developing melanoma too?

These questions usually trickle in when they are least expected, and the troubling thoughts can last for weeks or months. I tell my patients that this is a normal reaction because they have been actively engaged in learning about this disease. A diagnosis of melanoma changes an individual's attitude, behavior, and lifestyle. I call this second part of melanoma management the "marathon phase," reflecting the ongoing journey.

This chapter is divided into the following sections:

I. Medical Follow-Up
II. How Does a Dermatologist Find a New Melanoma?
III. How Can You Find a New Melanoma?
IV. How to Prevent Melanoma
V. Why You Should Not Use Tanning Beds
VI. Who Else in My Family Is at Risk for Developing Melanoma?
VII. Technological Innovations

I. Medical Follow-Up

Why Do You Need Continual Follow-Up?

The benefit of medical follow-up immediately following surgery or other treatments is obvious. Your physicians want to make sure that the surgical scar is healing well, that you have recovered fully from the treatment, and that you do not have any major side effects from it. What is not clear to some patients is why they need ongoing follow-up for years to come.

There are two major reasons for long-term follow-up. First, you need to make sure that the original melanoma has not come back. For patients who had intermediate (stage II) or advanced stages (stages III or IV) of melanoma, continual follow-up is needed to make certain that the melanoma has not spread to other body parts. In those cases, a medical history, physical examination, and laboratory and imaging studies may be ordered to monitor your health.

When Do Melanomas Usually Recur?

Here is a good place to answer the common question about the probability of recurrence. In general, early-stage melanomas recur very infrequently. If they do recur, they tend to come back after an extended period. In contrast, late-stage melanomas recur more often and more quickly. The risk of recurrence generally decreases over time, peaking at a rate between 2 and 5 percent, but it never gets down to zero. One study showed that 80 percent of all recurrences for stage I melanoma occurred within the first three years of diagnosis. Another study showed that the risk of recurrence reached a low level around four years after initial treatment for patients with stage I or II melanomas. Surprisingly, studies have shown that patients with stage III melanoma have their risk of recurrence reach a very low level at 2.7 years after initial treatment. Often clinicians use the five-year mark as a milestone, as the risk of recurrence dramatically decreases five years after the treatment of melanoma.

What Do Physicians Look For to Tell If a Melanoma Is Coming Back or Has Spread Elsewhere?

How physicians check for recurrence or metastasis is another question on the minds of many patients who have had melanoma. Your physician will pay special attention to the surgical scar, looking for any new pigmentation developing within or extending beyond the scar. You physician will also feel (palpate) the scar, checking for any underlying bumps, nodules, or firm lesions in or around the scar. All this visual and tactile inspection is done to detect any recurrent melanomas located near the surgical site.

To look for distant spread, your physician will palpate the lymph nodes in your groin, armpits, and around the neck to make sure that melanoma has not spread to them. Depending on the stage of the initial melanoma, your physician may order imaging studies, such as a CT or PET scan, to make sure no melanoma appears in distant organs.

What Is My Risk of Getting Another Melanoma?

The second reason for having follow-ups is that they provide an opportunity to detect any new melanoma at an early stage. People with a personal history of melanoma are at a higher risk for developing new melanoma, especially in the five years after being diagnosed with the first one. It is estimated that 2 to 10 percent of patients with one melanoma later develop a second one. Approximately 30 percent of all second melanomas are diagnosed at the same time or within the first three months after the initial melanoma was diagnosed. Approximately 50 percent of second melanomas are diagnosed within the first year. Second melanomas are likely to occur in the same anatomic region as the first one. For example, if the first melanoma occurred on the back, then a second melanoma is usually located on the back too. The explanation for this is that this region of the body received a similar amount of ultraviolet damage from the sun. Hence it is important to examine that region with particular care.

The statistics are more alarming for patients with two melanomas. The risk of developing a third melanoma is estimated to be 16 percent by one year and 30 percent by five years. There is some good news, however. Studies have shown that subsequent melanomas usually have less Breslow thickness than the initial melanoma. For example, if the first melanoma has a Breslow thickness of 1.2 mm, the second one may be only 0.5 mm. This favorable early detection of a subsequent melanoma is largely attributed to vigilant surveillance. That is, frequent skin examination by a dermatologist and self-examination by the patient have been identified as the reason for diagnosing a new melanoma at an earlier stage.

What Specialist or Specialists Should You See for Follow-Ups?

The answer to this question about what specialist to see depends on the stage of your melanoma. Patients with early stages (e.g., stage I) of melanoma may only need to have their dermatologist conduct a total-body skin examination looking for new skin cancers. For these patients, the role of medical oncologists and surgeons may be limited, and some melanoma patients may never need follow-up care from these other specialists.

For patients who had an intermediate (e.g., stage II) or advanced stage (e.g., stage III or IV) of the disease, medical oncologists and surgeons will have a larger role in follow-up. Surgeons will focus on the scar, check the lymph nodes, and regard other surgery-related issues. Medical oncologists and internists tend to focus on overall health status and make sure that the melanoma has not recurred or spread to other parts of the body.

How Frequently Should You Have Follow-Up Exams?

The National Comprehensive Cancer Network Guidelines have recommendations for the frequency of clinical follow-up. The frequency depends on the stage of the disease and the number of years that have passed since the initial diagnosis. Patients with advanced stage melanoma need to have much more frequent follow-ups. Patients whose diagnosis and treatment were recent also need to have more frequent follow-ups. As a general rule, patients with a history of melanoma should be seen by a physician at least once a year. For more details, please see the description below on the follow-up schedule according to the stage of melanoma (page 78).

What Should You Expect during Follow-Up Visits?

At follow-up visits, your physicians will ask about your overall health, current medications, and the status of any other medical conditions. Specifically, they may ask about any weight loss, weight gain, or symptoms associated with particular organs. These questions elicit information related to the history of present illness, a review of systems, and past medical history.

Asking such questions is the initial screening tool for physicians checking to see whether melanoma has spread to any distant organ. For example, patients with a persistent cough may prompt a suspicion that melanoma has spread to the lungs, especially if the patient has no other symptoms of the flu or a cold such as a runny nose or fever. In this case, further workup with imaging studies may be warranted to test the clinical suspicion.

In addition to taking a patient's history and asking questions, physicians will perform a physical examination. The scope of the examination will vary depending on the specialist you are seeing. For example, dermatologists will check the skin by performing a total-body skin examination, including the scalp and the bottoms of your feet. They will attend in particular to melanoma surgical scars, looking for signs of recurrence at the original surgical site. Medical oncologists and general internists may listen to your lungs, heart, and abdomen with a stethoscope, and they may palpate your abdomen to check for any potential enlargement of your liver or spleen.

Putting it all together, the following is an outline of the frequency and type of follow-ups recommended for patients with different stages of melanoma. Please see chapter 2 if you need to review staging definitions. The recommendations below largely come from the National Comprehensive Cancer Network Guidelines. *The information below* **cannot**, *however, cover the nuances associated with all types of follow-up for various stages of melanomas. It* **does not** *replace the advice and treatment plans offered by your own doctors.*

Stage 0 (melanoma in situ or lentigo maligna). Patients are recommended to have at least one skin check annually. Routine blood tests to screen for local, regional, or distant metastasis are not recommended. In addition, any routine imaging studies, such as a CT or PET scan, to screen for local or regional recurrence or for distant metastasis are not recommended unless patients have associated symptoms.

Stages IA to IIA. Patients are recommended to have a skin exam once every 6 to 12 months for the first five years. Afterwards, an annual follow-up exam is recommended. Again, routine blood tests to screen for local or regional recurrence or for distant metastasis are not recommended. If patients do not have any suspicious symptoms, imaging studies to screen for local or regional recurrence or for distant metastasis are not recommended.

Stages IIB to IV. Patients are recommended to have skin exams every 3–6 months for the first two years and then every 3–12 months for the next three years. Afterwards, an annual follow-up exam is recommended. Imaging studies are recommended to investigate any specific signs or symptoms. Routine imaging may be needed for patients with stage III or IV melanoma in certain cases to screen for local or regional recurrence or for distant metastasis.

Again, these guidelines are generalized recommendations. Your physicians may deviate from them. For example, your dermatologist may see you every three months even if you only had stage IA disease, especially if you have had multiple melanomas and numerous atypical nevi (moles).

What Can I Do to Improve the Appearance of My Scar

I want to discuss briefly surgical scars. Unfortunately, scarring is an unavoidable side effect of melanoma treatment. There are several factors that influence the final appearance of a scar: the patient's age and race, the anatomic site, the size and depth of the initial melanoma, the surgeon's skill, and even luck (believe it or not). In general, scars on the trunk and legs do not heal as well as scars on the face and arms. Compared with young patients, older patients tend to have less visible scars in the long run.

Individuals who are prone to get hypertrophic scars or keloids will have more visible scars.

There are a number of precautions and aftercare measures you can take to achieve better outcomes for scars. In the immediate period of 7 to 14 days after surgery, avoid strenuous activities and exercises by allowing the wound to heal. Physical activities may increase the risk of infection or sutures bursting open; both are complications that will slow wound healing and can result in more noticeable scars. During this period, keep the surgical site moist with Vaseline or Aquaphor ointment. Dried or scabbed wounds take longer to heal.

Scars tend to fade over time. In fact, there is a great deal of truth in the phrase "a tincture of time heals all wounds." I tell my patients that it will take at least six months for a scar to attain its final shape, color, and texture. There are some special gels and silicon sheets that can improve the appearance of scars, but in most cases, they are not necessary.

In certain cases, patients need interventions to improve the appearance of scars. Some of the modalities include injectable steroids, additional surgery, and laser treatment. For more information on how to correct scars, please watch my interview with **Dr. Deborah Sarnoff** (https://www .beatingmelanoma.com/deborah-s -sarnoff), who is a dermatologist and cosmetic surgeon.

1. Scan the code
2. Find the expert
3. Watch the interview

II. How Does a Dermatologist Find a New Melanoma?

You should schedule a total-body skin examination with your physician, preferably with a dermatologist. Dermatologists are by far the best-trained and most-skilled physicians at diagnosing melanomas and non-melanoma skin cancers. Among dermatologists, there are those who have more expertise because they focus only on diagnosing and treating skin cancers, especially melanomas. These expert dermatologists tend not to see patients with general skin conditions (e.g., acne, eczema, or psoriasis) or with cosmetic concerns (e.g., Botox or filler injection or laser treatment). These skin cancer experts have higher diagnostic accuracy; they are better at avoiding over- or under-diagnosing melanoma or other skin cancers.

Below is a description of what I and other melanoma specialists do in our practice. In general, we have two goals: (1) diagnosing melanoma as early as possible and (2) avoiding unnecessary skin biopsies that will scar patients. Many melanoma patients complain that they always get a few skin biopsies every time they see their physician. In most cases, the biopsies are benign, and patients are left with multiple scars. One of my patients described himself as looking like Swiss cheese after having 30 skin biopsies performed by other physicians.

Total-Body Skin Exam

A total-body skin exam is the first line of defense. The reason is simple: melanoma can occur almost *anywhere* on the skin. In order to detect it, we need to look for it everywhere.

I take every possible measure to respect the comfort, privacy, and modesty of my patients. My staff asks patients to remove all clothing except for underwear. Women have the option of removing or keeping on their bra. We provide a gown. Personally, I prefer using a regular gown, not the paper type, as they provide more comfort and privacy for patients.

If a patient complains of feeling cold, our staff offers a warm blanket or increases the temperature in the exam room. Before conducting the skin exam, I usually inquire about the patient's overall health and make sure there are no suspicious signs or symptoms suggesting that melanoma may have spread to other parts of the body. I also like to chat with patients to find out what else is going on with their personal, family, and work life. These conversations may cover their kids, parents, work, or recent vacations. To me, getting to know my patients is the most enjoyable part of being a physician. During these conversations, I get to learn about the world and life and hear interesting or funny anecdotes. A side benefit of these casual, sometimes intimate, conversations is that my patients are more relaxed and less anxious.

My students and residents ask me why it matters whether a patient has a relaxed mindset. My answer is that coming to a cancer center for care is stressful. Fear may prompt some patients to skip, deliberately or unconsciously, their annual follow-up. In addition, I like to educate patients during the exam. When stressed, patients may not comprehend or remember what I tell them. These conversations help to build rapport and trust. Trust between a patient and a physician is sacred and essential. Without trust, there will be no compliance. Without compliance, patients will not follow my treatment plan, and they will not get well.

Next comes the exam. I always follow a routine for a skin exam. I like to exam parts of the body in the same sequence. It helps me be consistent and avoid skipping any parts.

I start by looking at the patient's right hand and move up to the right arm. I then focus on the back and shift to the left arm and then the left hand. Next, I examine the chest and abdomen. After the upper body, I turn my attention to the thighs, lower legs, feet (both top and bottom), toe webs, and toenails. The last stop is the face and the scalp, making sure that no skin cancers are hiding in the hair. Once I finish the skin exam, I put on my gloves and feel the groin, armpits, and head and neck area to check the lymph nodes. I do not routinely examine the genital area unless the patient requests an examination there or we are monitoring moles there. One reason I do not routinely examine the genital area is that the incidence of melanoma and other skin cancer in the genital area is exceedingly low. In addition, many patients feel uncomfortable about it. I do, however, commonly ask patients if they have any concerns about areas that are covered by underwear.

You may ask, What am I looking for? How do I know which lesions are benign or malignant? These are not easy questions to answer. I rely on the following principles during a clinical exam.

The ABCDE Rule

The ABCDE rule is a memory aid created by melanoma specialists at New York University's medical center more than 20 years ago. *A* stands for **a**symmetry, *B* for **b**order irregularity, *C* for multiple **c**olors, *D* for **d**iameter greater than 6 mm, and *E* for **e**volution or change. The purpose of this mnemonic is to highlight the features of melanomas visible to the naked eye and so help physicians and the public spot this skin cancer at an early stage. Originally, *E* (evolution) was not included, but now evolution is considered to be an important feature. Table 3.1 spells out the system, and figure 3.1 gives some examples. The ABCDE rule is useful for detecting obvious melanomas, but it is not very useful for detecting early melanomas. In my clinical practice, most of the melanomas I find lack the ABCDE features. For more about the ABCDE rule, please watch my interview with **Dr. Darrell Rigel** (https://www .beatingmelanoma.com/darrell-s -rigel), who was one of the authors who first publicized the rule.

1. Scan the code
2. Find the expert
3. Watch the interview

Table 3.1. The ABCDE Rule for Monitoring Lesions

A stands for *a*symmetry of the lesion. This criterion considers the shape of the lesion. If a lesion could fold in on itself in two directions without overlap, it is said to be symmetrical along two axes. In general, *a*symmetrical lesions are worrisome.

B stands for *b*order irregularities. In general, lesions with irregular (not smooth) borders are worrisome.

C stands for multiple *c*olors. In general, lesions with many colors are a cause for concern.

D stands for *d*iameter of the lesion greater than 6 mm, which is about the size of a pencil's eraser.

E stands for *e*volution, or change, in the shape, color, size, or symptoms of the lesion.

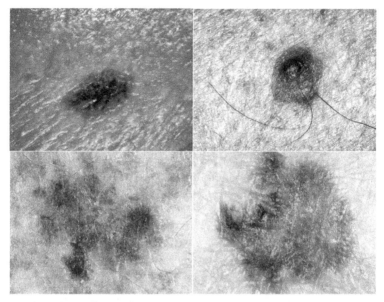

Figure 3.1. Melanomas can appear in a wide variety of shape, color, and size. Each of these four photos shows the ABCDE features of melanomas.

Ugly Duckling Sign

The "ugly duckling" sign refers to a lesion (irregular spot) on the skin that does not have the same appearance as other moles nearby (figure 3.2). This sign has been demonstrated to be a very effective way of identifying melanomas. During my exams, I first scan an anatomic region as a whole (e.g., the whole right arm or the whole back), looking for any lesion that stands out or looks different from its neighboring moles. An ugly duckling mole may be darker or lighter in color than surrounding moles, or it may just be larger. A mole that stands out is a suspicious one and warrants closer inspection with additional tools, such as a dermatoscope.

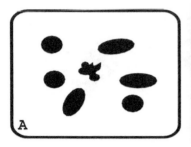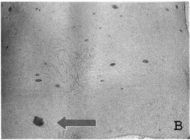

Figure 3.2. The "ugly duckling sign" refers to a lesion that looks different from its neighbors. (A) Drawn illustration. (B) Photograph of a large atypical lesion (*arrow*) that looks different from neighboring moles.

Symptomatic Lesions

I pay attention to *lesions with symptoms*. One of the questions I routinely ask patients before conducting an exam is "Do you have any lesions with symptoms of pain, itching, or bleeding?" In addition, I usually inquire if the patient has noticed any lesions that have changed in shape, color, or size since the last skin exam. A lesion with symptoms or changes is not necessarily a malignant lesion; in my mind, it simply means that I should look at that lesion more closely.

Dermoscopy Exam

No skin exam is complete without looking at almost every single lesion on the body with a dermatoscope. A dermatoscope is a handheld microscope-like device (figure 3.3) that allows a clinician to see the structures of lesions below the skin surface. Normally, these structures are not visible to the naked eye.

A dermatoscope is a small and simple device, but interpreting what one sees under it takes experience and

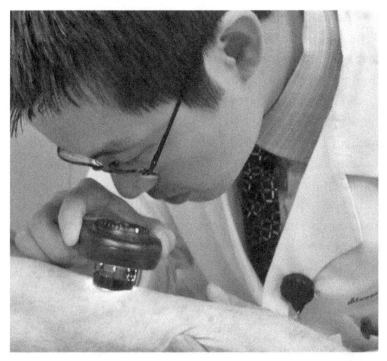

Figure 3.3. A dermatoscope in use during a skin examination.

knowledge. In the hands of experts, dermoscopy can significantly increase the accuracy and confidence of melanoma diagnosis. Training and experience are crucial, though. Studies have shown that diagnostic accuracy for beginners when using a dermatoscope is actually worse than when using the naked eye alone because some over-diagnosis tends to occur. Over time, and with training, accuracy in using a dermatoscope rapidly increases.

Many lesions can appear worrisome on a naked eye exam that will appear completely normal or benign under dermoscopic examination. Using the dermatoscope, I can reassure my patients with complete confidence that lesions are totally normal. More importantly, dermoscopy helps me find many early melanomas and early non-melanoma skin cancers that I would have missed. These early melanomas are the ones that have no symptoms, no history of changes, and none of the ABCDE features.

Aside from improving the accuracy and confidence of my diagnosis, a dermoscopic examination also helps me predict whether a suspicious lesion is an early- or late-stage melanoma. I can predict with relative certainty when a lesion is a melanoma in situ versus just an atypical mole with moderate or severe atypia. Depending on what I see under the dermatoscope, I can plan different biopsy techniques to remove the lesion, plan definitive treatment options, and schedule a surgical appointment depending on the urgency. All of this extra information is valuable. I can communicate my prediction to my patients at the time of biopsy and prepare them mentally for what may come next.

The dermatoscope has become the stethoscope for a dermatologist. My colleagues and I rely on this simple tool so much that we find it difficult to do our job without it. On rare occasions, when my dermatoscope runs out of battery power, I have to apologize to my patients, recharge my dermatoscope, and then resume the exam.

Total-Body Photography

Total-body photography is another tool that has improved dermatologists' ability to detect skin cancer at an early stage and to avoid unnecessary biopsy. Many of my patients are at very high risk for developing melanoma. They may have more than 100 moles, and many of them look like melanoma. They are asymmetric in shape, have irregular borders, are larger than 6 mm, and have multiple colors. Some of these lesions even have a history of changes in size, shape, or color. In other words, they display most, if not all, of the ABCDE criteria of melanoma and are causes for concern. Some of these patients also have a personal and family history of melanoma, both of which are risk factors for developing melanoma. Total-body photography is extremely helpful in keeping track of all these worrisome moles.

In total-body photography, a set of baseline digital photographs of the entire body's surface is taken by a professional medical photographer. The high-resolution digital photographs are stored on a secure computer server or cloud server. At each visit, as I perform the skin exam, I bring up these digital photos on the computer screen and compare the moles on the patient with the digital photos. Total-body photographs make it possible to track changes in the moles from that baseline set of appearances. Using this type of tracking system, we can detect minute changes and spot new moles.

Total-body photographs can also be a useful tool for patients when they perform self-exams. In the past, patients would receive a large book of color prints and a CD containing digital copies of their total-body photographs. More recently these photos are stored on a secure cloud server, and patients are given an access code and follow a two-step authentication steps to pull up these photos at home. They can have these digital photos displayed on their desktop, laptop, or iPad during their self-exams and compare the baseline pictures with the current appearance of their moles.

Recently, a number of medical centers have acquired a cutting-edge photographic system called Canfield Vectra

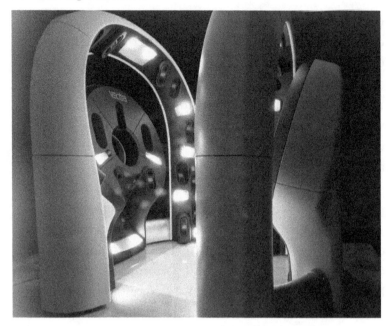

Figure 3.4. Photo of the Vectra WB360 imaging system.

WB360 3D Total Body Photography (figure 3.4). It has a number of distinct advantages over conventional photography. The Vectra 360 system uses 92 high-resolution cameras that fire simultaneously to capture the whole body in less than a second. It is super fast, so patients no longer have to stand in front of a photographer for a photo session. Most patients feel somewhat embarrassed standing naked in front a stranger, albeit medical personnel, for over 30 minutes.

Once the photos are taken, software "stiches" all the images together and creates a high-resolution 3D avatar of the body. These 3D digital photos are more accurate for comparison when we want to detect new lesions or track lesions with small changes. The software also has a number of highly sophisticated features that can automatically select the most suspicious lesions based on parameters set by the clinician. At some major academic institutions, melanoma experts have started to adopt this imaging system as the preferred standard.

For more information on photographic machinery, please watch my interview with **Dr. Allan Halpern** (https://www.beatingmelanoma.com/allan-c-halpern), who is a world expert on melanoma.

1. Scan the code
2. Find the expert
3. Watch the interview

Short-Term Follow-Up with Digital Photos

As I have said, accurate early detection and diagnosis, followed by prompt treatment, ensures the best clinical outcome. There are times, however, when it is simply not possible to know for sure whether a lesion is benign or malignant.

Patients are often perplexed when I try to explain this concept, but biology is not always clear-cut. Although many lesions can be clearly classified as benign or malignant, a number of lesions occupy a gray zone where their biological nature cannot be clearly determined at the time of the exam. Some of these concerning lesions may turn into a malignant lesion in the near or distant future, while others will never become malignant at all. At that particular stage in the lesion's life cycle, we simply cannot tell through clinical and dermoscopic exams. This is a limitation to the current state of diagnosing melanoma, and this limitation affects the best experts in the world.

Even when the biologic status of a lesion remains uncertain after visual examination, there are clinical scenarios where biopsy may not be desired or even possible for various reasons. For example, a young woman may not be inclined to have a lesion on her face or chest biopsied because it would leave a scar in a cosmetically sensitive area.

When faced with this kind of challenge, I often rely on sequential short-term monitoring for worrisome moles. Rather than performing a biopsy, I take close-up clinical and dermoscopic photos of the concerning lesions. Then, I have the patient return in three months. I reexamine the lesions and take another set of close-up clinical and dermoscopic photos of them for comparison. The images are displayed on a high-resolution monitor, and I look for any differences between the two sets of images. If I do not see changes, I usually do not recommend biopsy and proceed with ongoing follow-up. If there are significant changes over the interval period, I biopsy the lesion to rule out melanoma. This approach to monitoring is reserved for special circumstances.

You may wonder whether this approach can potentially delay diagnosis and lead to an unfavorable prognosis. The answer is generally no for the following reasons. First, we dermatologists have the patient return in three months, a short interval time, for follow-up. Second, we select only a certain type of lesion for short-term monitoring. These lesions are usually flat ones. Even if they have the potential to be melanoma, studies have shown that this type of lesion grows very slowly. A three-month delay does not alter the prognosis. It is paramount to mention that we never use this short-term monitoring technique to follow raised lesions, because this type of melanoma can grow very fast. What is more, I have to know and trust that the patient will be compliant and return in three months for follow-up.

Confocal Laser Microscopy

A confocal laser microscope is an imaging device designed to examine skin tissue in a noninvasive fashion. The benefit to this imaging technique is that doctors can see cellular detail without taking a lesion biopsy. Similar to X-ray, MRI, and CT imaging used to see internal organs, a confocal laser microscope delivers high-resolution images of skin, showing in rich detail the individual skin cells and their nuclei. The high resolution of a confocal image can even reveal red blood cells tumbling through blood vessels.

The clarity and magnification of confocal laser microscopy is comparable to that of standard microscopes. Aside from the noninvasive nature and high-resolution imaging of the device, an additional advantage is that a confocal laser microscope can examine the skin tissue layer by layer. By adjusting the focal plane of the device, a physician can selectively look at the layer of skin of most interest.

Confocal laser microscopy has been refined and improved since it was introduced into the clinical setting as a research tool in the 1980s. It has transitioned from a tool used purely for research purposes into a tool used in patient care. It is valuable for diagnosing lentigo melanoma, a type of melanoma in situ commonly found on the face. Differentiating lentigo maligna from other benign skin lesions, such as solar lentigo, atypical nevi, and pigmented actinic keratosis, is quite difficult, even with the use of a dermatoscope. By using confocal laser microscopy, physicians can usually decide whether a lesion on the face needs a biopsy. More importantly, the device can guide physicians to decide where to biopsy in a lesion.

Despite its potential, confocal laser microscopy has
limitations. It is time consuming to image a lesion. The
device is expense, and extensive training is needed to
master the interpretation of images obtained from a confocal laser microscope. For these reasons, this technology is
still not widely adopted. For more detail on confocal laser
microscopy, please watch my interview with my colleague
Dr. Harold Rabinovitz (https://www.beatingmelanoma
.com/harold-rabinovitz), who is a
dermatologist and world expert on
confocal laser microscopy.

1. Scan the code
2. Find the expert
3. Watch the interview

Total-body skin exam, dermoscopy, total-body photographs, short-term monitoring, and confocal laser microscopy provide a powerful combination of tools for detecting
melanomas. One significant advantage of such careful
monitoring is that it reduces unnecessary biopsies of
benign (normal) lesions. The efficacy of these tools has
been studied well in Europe, Australia, and the United
States. Let me clarify, though, that these tools do not
replace skin biopsy. Instead, they increase diagnostic
accuracy and work especially well with high-risk melanoma patients.

For more details on how physicians diagnose melanomas while avoiding unnecessary biopsies, please watch
my interviews with the following dermatologists and
melanoma experts: **Dr. David Swanson** (https://www
.beatingmelanoma.com/david-swanson), **Dr. Harold Rabinovitz** (https://www.beatingmelanoma.com/harold
-rabinovitz), **Dr. Allan Halpern** (https://www.beatingmela
noma.com/allan-c-halpern), **Dr. Trilokraj Tejasvi**
(https://www.beatingmelanoma.com/trilokraj-tejasvi),

Dr. David Polsky (https://www.beatingmelanoma.com
/david-polsky), and **Dr. Justin Ko**
(https://www.beatingmelanoma
.com/justin-ko).

1. Scan the code
2. Find the expert
3. Watch the interview

Biopsy Plus Pathology, the Gold Standard

The clinical approaches and technological tools I have
described correspond with a philosophy for managing
patients with melanoma: early detection is key while
avoiding unnecessary biopsy. Of course, biopsy is often
unavoidable and the only way to make a definitive diagnosis. Below I describe different types of skin biopsies.

The most common type is the shave biopsy. After
numbing the lesion and surrounding area with lidocaine, I
simply shave a thin slice from the worrisome lesion with a
razor blade–like instrument. In this procedure, no sutures
(stitches) are used to close the wound. Any bleeding is
stopped either with cautery (burning) or aluminum
chloride solution. A small dab of Vaseline or Aquaphor
ointment is applied to the wound, and a bandage covers it.

Another common technique is called punch biopsy.
With a pencil-shaped device, much like a tiny cookie
cutter, a lesion is "punched," or cut out. Sutures are usually used to close the wound after a punch biopsy. A small
dab of Vaseline or Aquaphor ointment is applied to the
wound, and a bandage covers it. The patient may need to
return in one to two weeks for suture removal depending
on the location and type of suture used.

The final type of is called excisional biopsy. This
method is more involved and is used to biopsy a large
lesion. An elliptical, or football-shaped, section of skin is

removed with a scalpel that contains a surgical blade. Any bleeding is stopped with cautery. The wound is closed usually with multiple layers of sutures, and a pressure bandage dressing is applied to the wound. Depending on the suture used, the patient may need to return in one to two weeks for suture removal.

These different techniques of biopsy are chosen according to the size of the lesion, its location on the body, and even the physician's surgical expertise. Regardless of the technique, here are a few tenets of quality biopsy.

First, if possible, your physician should biopsy the entire lesion, not a portion of the lesion. Partial biopsies may miss the diagnosis of melanoma and misjudge the Breslow thickness of the melanoma owing to sampling error.

Second, the biopsy must reach an adequate depth in the skin, especially if there is any concern that the lesion is a melanoma. It is critical that tissue is taken deeply enough to determine the correct Breslow thickness, as this measure is needed to decide on an optimal treatment plan. I have consulted with numerous patients who had biopsies taken at other institutions where the pathology report mentioned that the melanoma was only partially transected (i.e., was not biopsied deeply enough).

Fortunately, in most cases, a shallow biopsy does not change the management plan that much. However, if a patient has melanoma with a Breslow thickness of 0.8 mm without ulceration, but the base of the lesion is not transected, then the inadequate biopsy in this case will pose a quandary for management decisions. The criterion for recommending sentinel lymph node biopsy is any melanoma with Breslow thickness > 1 mm. When a biopsy is not deep enough (i.e., where the melanoma is not transected at its base), it is impossible to know the melanoma's true depth. In those cases, your physician will need a lengthy discussion to explain the issue and to decide if sentinel lymph node biopsy should be performed or not.

Third, if a lesion is too large to be removed or biopsied in its entirety, your physician may consider taking a biopsy of the most worrisome portion of the lesion as seen with a dermatoscope. In some cases, the physician may need to take multiple samples from different locations of a large lesion.

Before ending this section on biopsy, I offer one more piece of advice. If you have a biopsy done, you should take a photo of the biopsied site with your phone following the procedure. As part of your treatment, your dermatologist may refer you to a dermatologic or oncologic surgeon to operate on the melanoma. Because you will be seeing someone who did not perform the biopsy, the surgeon will need to verify its exact location. The pathology report names the general body part (e.g., left abdomen) but not the lesion's exact location. Studies have shown that it is not uncommon for both patients and physicians to be unable to identify a biopsy site reliably at a later time, especially after the biopsy scar has healed. If you take a photo of the site immediately after the biopsy, you can later show it to the surgeon on your phone. This simple trick avoids the potential for a surgeon to operate on the wrong lesion.

III. How Can You Find a New Melanoma?

Physicians, especially dermatologists, play an important role in finding any new melanoma, but many clinical studies have shown that most melanomas are first spotted by the patients or their family members or friends. Hence, *you* can detect melanomas on yourself and on your friends and family members. A significant proportion of all melanomas are brought to a physician's attention by the patients themselves. Some studies have estimated that nearly 75 percent of new melanomas are found by patients, their friends, or their family members.

Perform Regular Self-Exams of Your Skin

Routinely self-examining your skin is crucial. People with a personal history of melanoma have a higher risk of developing subsequent melanomas and other skin cancers than the general population. The risk of developing new lesions, or of having the original melanoma come back, is especially high in the first five years after the initial melanoma diagnosis. That is why patients need to perform skin exams on themselves once a month, *every month*.

Let me describe how to perform a self-exam of your skin. Standing in front of a full-length mirror, examine the front and both sides of your body with your arms raised. Look at your forearms, underarms, and hands. Use a handheld mirror to check your back and buttocks. Moving downward, examine your legs and feet. Spread your toes and look at the skin between them. Don't forget to look at the bottom of your feet. You will need the handheld mirror to examine your neck and scalp. For the scalp and back, consider asking your spouse, a close friend, or a family member to help you examine them.

Patients often ask, "What should I look for?" or "What are the clues of melanoma?" They want to perform self-examinations, but they have no idea what they should be looking for. I can certainly empathize with their concern because accurately diagnosing melanoma is not easy. It is difficult even for dermatologists. You can improve your ability to spot worrisome lesions by following these simple strategies.

Remember the ABCDE rule. To repeat the mnemonic: *A* stands for *asymmetry, B* for *border* irregularity, *C* for multiple *colors, D* for *diameter* greater than 6 mm, and *E* for *evolution* or change. Although I do not find this rule to be especially helpful in my clinical practice, it is very useful for the general public in spotting worrisome lesions. Among the five criteria, I instruct my patients to pay more attention to evolution. Any changing lesions should be examined more closely or brought to the attention of a dermatologist.

Look for the "ugly duckling" sign. As a reminder, this term refers to a lesion on the skin that does not have the same appearance as other moles on the surrounding skin (figure 3.2). This simple method is surprisingly effective in finding melanomas.

Pay attention to symptoms. Give extra attention to any moles or lesions that are painful, itching, or bleeding and any that have changed in shape, color, or size since you last examined your skin. Show your physician these moles or lesions. Other skin cancers, including basal cell carcinoma (BCC) and squamous cell carcinoma (SCC) have similar symptoms, and both SCC and BCC are far more common than melanoma; your examinations may help detect these as well. (Appendixes A and B describe these two other types of skin cancer.)

These three strategies—the ABCDE rule, the ugly duckling sign, and paying attention to symptoms—work well for detecting worrisome lesions. Do not be concerned if you find it difficult when you first start performing self-exams. Many of my patients tell me that they do not know if they are doing the exam correctly. Some patients stop doing their skin exams because they have so many doubts about what they are seeing, or they become anxious about every little spot. I tell them that the purpose of performing self-exams is not to train themselves to diagnose skin cancers. They are not expected to achieve a high diagnostic accuracy when it comes to spotting early melanoma.

Instead, the goal of skin self-examination is for you and anyone who helps you to become familiar with your moles and lesions. You are looking for *changes and symptoms.* You are providing another pair of eyes to help your doctor spot worrisome lesions. If you find some moles or lesions that are concerning to you, consult your physician. Do not wait. Over time you will get better at distinguishing benign lesions from worrisome ones. A few of my vigilant high-risk patients have become rather good at spotting worrisome lesions over the years.

In addition to helping detect early melanomas, another benefit of skin self-exam is that doing it routinely prompts you to practice other behaviors that can prevent skin cancer. Doing these monthly exams will remind you to avoid excessive ultraviolet exposure, wear protective clothing, and apply sunscreen on a daily basis. The aim is to reinforce long-term, consistent behavior modification, much like the way that maintaining an exercise regimen helps people watch their diet: the act of daily exercise motivates them to follow an overall healthy lifestyle.

IV. How to Prevent Melanoma

This is a perfect segue to discussing different strategies for preventing melanoma and other types of skin cancer. There is an entire science focused on *primary prevention*: the strategy of helping people not develop melanoma in the first place. Primary prevention involves changing a person's perception and behavior with regard to ultraviolet exposure from the sun or any artificial UV sources (e.g., tanning beds). You cannot control your family history, your skin type, or moles present at birth, but you can exert considerable control over your exposure to UV radiation from the sun or other sources. Many scientific studies have demonstrated that intermittent and intense sun exposure plays a major role in the development of melanoma. Hence, anything you can do to reduce harmful UV exposure may help you prevent skin cancer.

Primary Prevention: Avoid Excessive Exposure to Ultraviolet Light

The main goal of primary prevention is to reduce your overall exposure to ultraviolet radiation, whether it comes from the sun or from any other source, such as a tanning booth. Here are five steps to protecting yourself, ranked in order of importance:

1. Avoid excessive sun exposure and stay away from tanning booths.
2. Seek shade.
3. Wear protective clothing, hats, and sunglasses.
4. Use sunscreen.
5. Take oral supplements.

Avoiding the sun. Staying out of the sun is the best way to reduce UV exposure. Total avoidance is not possible, of course, and may even be detrimental to our health. There are some health benefits associated with sun exposure. Outdoor activities promote an active and healthy lifestyle. Sunshine also brightens our mood. Many patients tell me, "Dr. Wang, I like being in the sun. It actually makes me feel good." Recent scientific studies have confirmed that these subjective feelings of mood enhancement are based on biology

UV radiation, however, induces DNA damage to skin cells. As a response, the melanocytes, specialized cells in the skin, produce and transport the skin pigment melanin to shield the DNA of the skin cells. Think of melanin as the body's natural sunscreen to block UV rays. The biologic signal that triggers the production of melanin also induces the release of endorphin, a feel-good chemical that brightens one's mood. The release of endorphin is the biological explanation for why many patients feel happier after UV exposure. To learn more about the complex biology of melanin, please watch my interview with **Dr. David Fisher** (https://www.beatingmelanoma.com /david-fisher).

1. Scan the code
2. Find the expert
3. Watch the interview

Complete sun avoidance is not possible and not recommended. You should not feel guilty the next time you are out in the sun. Just use commonsense precautions. Strive to cut back on the total amount of UV exposure, and try to avoid the peak UV radiation hours from 10 A.M. to 4 P.M. when UV rays are most intense.

Seeking shade. Whenever you are sitting or lying outdoors for an extended period, seek the shade provided by awnings, trees, or umbrellas. Staying in the shade allows you to enjoy being outdoors while still getting much of the protection you need from UV radiation.

Wearing hats, clothing, and sunglasses. In addition to avoiding the most intense rays of the sun and seeking shade, I advise my patients to wear UV-protective clothing and hats whenever they are staying outdoors for a prolonged period of time. Hats and full-coverage clothing have a number of advantages over sunscreen. They provide uniform protection from both UVA (i.e., long-range UV rays measuring from 320 nm to 400 nm) and UVB (i.e., short-range UV rays measuring from 290 nm to 320 nm). Most sunscreens available in the United States deliver more UVB protection than UVA protection. By comparison, clothing and hats offer more reliable protection as long as you remember to wear them. Also, clothing and hats are less costly than sunscreen over the long run. You should wear a hat with a wide brim all the way around to shades your ears, cheeks, nose, and the back of your neck. A baseball cap does not provide adequate shade, and UV rays penetrate the holes in a straw hat.

Some of my patients complain that long-sleeved shirts and pants are too hot to wear in the summer. Fortunately, an increasing number of specialty clothing manufacturers (e.g., Coolibar and Sun Precautions' Solumbra line) offer lightweight, breathable, and fashionable clothing designed to block UV rays from the sun. This clothing is made from special fabric with a close weave. These clothing lines satisfy everyone, including fashion-conscious individuals.

Aside from clothing and hats, always remember to wear sunglasses. Eyelid skin is very thin and especially vulnerable to UV ray damage. Although melanoma is not commonly found around eyelids, basal cell and squamous cell cancer are commonly found on the lower eyelids. In addition to skin cancer, UV rays can cause eye diseases, such as cataracts and pterygium. In general, most lenses are excellent at blocking out nearly all UVB and UVA rays. In terms of the shape of sunglasses, I recommend large lenses and a wraparound frame that cover the top, bottom, and sides of the eyes.

Applying sunscreen. In contrast to popular public perception, sunscreen should not be the first line of defense against UV rays. Sunscreen definitely helps to prevent skin cancers (e.g., melanoma), sunburn, and premature aging, if they are used properly along with other protective measures. A number of large prospective clinical trials from Australia have shown that daily use of sunscreen with an SPF (sun protection factor) of 16 prevents melanoma by nearly 50 percent and squamous cell cancer by 40 percent.

In these studies, patients in the control (placebo) group were still allowed to use sunscreen. The only difference between the control group and sunscreen group were that patients in the sunscreen group were given free sunscreen. Plus, the sunscreens used in the studies had an SPF of 16, which is low and does not offer adequate UVA protection. The sunscreens used in the studies degrade quickly when exposed to UV radiation and become ineffective. In view of these shortcomings, sunscreens available today have much higher SPF values (e.g., SPF 50) and have more advanced UVA filters that can withstand UV rays. Hence,

I believe sunscreens on the market today are far superior to the ones used in the studies, and their real protective effect against skin cancer is much greater than the findings reported in the studies.

So, what are the shortcomings of sunscreen? First, *most people do not use enough sunscreen to achieve desired protection.* SPF is the well-known measure used to rate the efficacy of any sunscreen. All sunscreen products have an SPF number, such as SPF 30 or SPF 55. Unfortunately, for most users, the actual degree of SPF protection provided is much less than that stated on the product label. For example, a sunscreen with an SPF of 30 may provide only SPF 10 in a real-life setting. How can this be?

The SPF value of a sunscreen product is measured in a laboratory using human subjects. In the tests, a concentration of 2 milligrams of sunscreen per square centimeter of skin is applied to each person's back. The test is then performed, and an SPF score is assigned to the product. For an average adult to apply that concentration of sunscreen (2 mg/cm^2) over the whole body, that person would need to use 1.4 ounces of sunscreen (the capacity of a shot glass) at each application. Since most sunscreens come in 6- to 8-ounce tubes or bottles, an average-sized adult using sunscreen over the entire body at the tested amount will use up a whole container of sunscreen in only three to five applications. We know full well, though, that a container of sunscreen may be used by a family of three or more people over the whole summer, and at summer's end, there may be plenty of sunscreen left over.

The bottom line is that most people use much less than the desired amount. Studies have shown that most people use a concentration of only 0.5 to 1 mg/cm^2 of sunscreen at each application (and some use less). That is one-quarter to one-half the amount they should be using. Hence, in real-life settings, the degree of SPF protection is dramatically lower than what is claimed on sunscreen packaging. That is why a sunscreen with an SPF of 30 may provide protection that is equivalent to an SPF as low as 10 in the real-life setting.

In addition, *most sunscreens on the market may not provide balanced UVA-UVB protection.* Although many brands claim that their products offer a broad spectrum of both UVB and UVA protection, the degree of UVA protection varies from one product to another. This shortcoming was especially acute prior to 2012. Currently, all sunscreens have to pass critical wavelength tests to claim broad-spectrum UV protection.

Unfortunately, compared with sunscreens sold abroad, sunscreens in the United States may provide lower UVA protection. US manufacturers of sunscreens do not have all the UV filters (e.g., chemicals capable of absorbing UV rays) that are available to manufacturers elsewhere. In essence, US manufacturers are working with fewer and less effective UV filters, thereby making domestic sunscreen products with lower UVA protection. To get around these technical challenges, US manufacturers have adopted various innovative ways to formulate products with higher UVA protection.

What is the problem with inadequate UVA protection from sunscreen? The most obvious problem is that you may use a sunscreen and believe you are well protected from the whole range of UV rays. In fact, though, you may be receiving good protection from UVB radiation and only limited protection from UVA rays. A sunscreen with a high SPF may prevent you from getting sunburned and thus give you a false sense of security, encouraging you to stay out in the sun longer. The end result is that you may unknowingly receive a disproportionally large amount of UVA rays. We know that both UVB and UVA rays can cause skin cancer.

Aside from these challenges, *there is a part of the body that needs UV protection yet is often ignored.* The scalp is one area that can receive excessive sun exposure. Individuals with thinning hair or no hair are especially vulnerable to sunburn and skin cancer on the head. In fact, 10 to 15 percent of all skin cancers are found on the head. Despite those alarming statistics, most people do not apply sunscreen to the scalp because most sunscreens are heavy and ruin their hairstyles. To change behavior and get more people to start applying sunscreen to the scalp, one company, Zenon Life (https://zenonlife.com/), has invented a three-in-one scalp and hair sunscreen. In addition to preventing sunburn and skin cancer, this sunscreen can also style and add volume to hair. It can nourish and strengthen hair with a rich mixture of amino acids, essential oils, and antioxidants. This product can improve scalp protection by letting it be part of an individual's grooming routine.

I would be remiss if I did not acknowledge that there are many controversies over sunscreen regarding safety and environmental concerns. However, I have spent the past 15 years studying this subject and have lectured on and written numerous publications on the topic. My own conclusion is that sunscreens are safe and effective at preventing skin cancers.

For more information on how to practice safe sun behavior, please watch my interview with **Dr. Henry Lim** (https://www.beatingmelanoma.com/henry-w-lim), who is a longtime collaborator and one of the most trusted authorities in the world on sunscreen and photoprotection. If you are interested in learning more about the facts and controversies surrounding sunscreens, please watch my interviews with two world expert on this topic, **Dr. Adam Friedman** (https://www.beatingmelanoma.com/adam-friedman) and **Dr. Darrell Rigel** (https://www.beatingmelanoma.com/darrell-s-rigel).

1. Scan the code
2. Find the expert
3. Watch the interview

In summary, sunscreen is one part of a sun protection routine. Sunscreen is effective and safe to use, despite its shortcomings. In large part, its weakness comes from inadequate application. Please visit BeatingMelanoma.com for specific sunscreen recommendations. See table 3.2 for instructions on applying sunscreen properly.

Taking oral supplements. Many natural supplements have been studied to evaluate their protective properties for sunburns and skin cancers. In most cases, these compounds are antioxidants that work to neutralize free radicals. Free radicals are unstable molecules that have been shown to damage cells. Some of the studied compounds include selenium, vitamin C, vitamin E, green tea polyphenols, genistein, caffeine, ferulic acids, and resveratrol. All of these compounds have shown efficacy when the studies were performed in animals, but they have not consistently been shown to prevent sunburn and definitely have not been proven to provide a benefit in preventing skin cancer.

Table 3.2. Instructions for Applying Sunscreen Properly

---

1. Apply sunscreen before you go outdoors, ideally 20 minutes prior. If you forget to put on sunscreen before going outdoors, apply it when you are outside. Take the sunscreen with you so that you can reapply it periodically. Applying sunscreen is important for everyone in the family, including mothers. Mothers are often the ones who remind their husbands to use sunscreen and who put sunscreen on their children. If you put sunscreen on everyone else *after* you are already outdoors, you may have already been exposed to the sun without any UV protection for 20 to 30 minutes.

2. Use a generous amount. For an average-sized adult, the appropriate amount is approximately 1.4 ounces, or the volume of a shot glass.

3. Reapply sunscreen generously and regularly while you remain outdoors. If you are sweating profusely or are in contact with water, reapply sunscreen at least every two hours.

4. Remember to use sunscreen every day, even when it is overcast. You should use a sunscreen with broad-spectrum UV coverage (of both UVB and UVA rays). UV exposure is the main agent for causing uneven pigmentation, or blotches, on the face, and it can degrade collagens in the skin, making it wrinkle and sag.

There are two other compounds worth mentioning because there are convincing clinical data demonstrating their efficacy in preventing sunburn and skin cancer in humans.

The first compound is niacinamide, or vitamin B3; it has been proven to reduce the risk of squamous cell cancer and actinic keratosis (a type of pre–skin cancer). Niacinamide is normally found in meat, fish, milk, and green vegetables. In one study published in the *New England Journal of Medicine* in 2015, researchers from Australia found that an intake of 500 mg of niacinamide twice a day reduced the development of new non-melanoma skin cancer by 23 percent over the course of a one-year period. In some earlier studies, niacinamide was also shown to reduce actinic keratosis. The exact mechanism for how it works to prevent skin cancer is not entirely clear. It is hypothesized that niacinamide boosts cellular energy production and helps cells repair their damaged DNA. Note that niacinamide is different from the vitamin niacin.

The second compound is an extract derived from *Polypodium leucotomos*, a tropical fern native to Central and South America. Traditionally, this plant has been used in folk medicine to treat various inflammatory skin diseases, such as psoriasis, eczema, and vitiligo. The plant is rich in polyphenols and potent antioxidants, compounds that confer its anti-inflammatory properties for the skin. Extensive laboratory and human studies have shown that extracts derived from *Polypodium leucotomos* decrease UV-induced damage for human skin. Specifically, people who took an oral extract of the plant had a reduced sunburn reaction after UV exposure. In addition, skin biopsies demonstrated that people who consumed the extract had a lower number of DNA mutations induced by sun exposure.

The protective benefits of the extract are attributed to its rich antioxidants. Unlike sunscreens that blocks UV rays from damaging the skin, *Polypodium* does not block or absorb UV radiation. Instead, the antioxidants in the plant neutralize free radicals generated by UV rays when reacting with various organelles and compounds in skin cells.

Several brands of supplement on the market contain this extract. However, the efficacy of each brand may vary significantly due to differences in processing the *Polypodium* plant. There may also be inconsistent potency across batches. This variation can change the quantity and quality of the extract in the product.

Heliocare is one brand that most dermatologists endorse. This brand is trusted by the dermatology community because a majority of the laboratory and clinical studies on the benefits of *Polypodium* were conducted by the company. To enjoy the protective benefit of *Polypodium*, people can take a 240 mg capsule every morning or a 240 mg capsule one hour before sun exposure.

To learn more about oral supplements, please watch my interview with **Dr. Henry Lim** (https://www.beatingmelanoma .com/henry-w-lim).

1. Scan the code
2. Find the expert
3. Watch the interview

V. Why You Should Not Use Tanning Beds

You should not use indoor tanning beds, period. They are bad for your health. The tanning industry markets their services by tapping into our society's misguided notion that tanned skin is attractive and sexy. They promote the idea that tanned skin is a sign of affluence.

The industry also tells potential customers about the supposed benefits of using tanning booths. Most of these so-called health benefits are false promises, however. For instance, tanning salons often tell their customers that a base tan will help to prevent sunburn. This message appeals to individuals planning vacations in sunny climates, but the truth is that the tan generated by artificial tanning provides a paltry SPF of 2 to 3. More importantly, current science tells us that a tan is the body's response to biological damage on a cellular level.

The tanning industry also promotes the notion that tanning increases vitamin D synthesis. The truth is that the light sources in a tanning booth mainly emit UVA light, while UVB rays are needed for vitamin D synthesis. Hence, tanning beds are not effective for producing vitamin D.

Artificial tanning is associated with the development of melanoma and other skin cancers. Tanning also accelerates the aging process. A few years ago, one of my dermatologist colleagues consulted with me on the case of a 24-year-old man. The patient had walked into my colleague's office and complained about diffuse reddish patches on his lower back. He confessed that he frequently visited a tanning salon. As my colleague examined those patches, he was initially perplexed. The diffuse and extensive nature of the rash was suggestive of psoriasis, but it was not typical psoriasis. As he looked closer, he noted blood vessels in some of these patches. He performed a biopsy on one of them. The result was rather surprising. It was a basal cell carcinoma, a common type of skin cancer. He then biopsied a few more patches; they were all basal cell carcinomas. This was a difficult case to manage. What should he do? What was the best way to treat these many areas of skin cancer on the young man's back? Multiple surgeries would be needed to remove all the skin cancers, and these procedures would leave many scars. After a lengthy discussion, my colleague decided to start the man on imiquimod, a topical drug approved to treat basal cell cancer. Most of the skin cancers were successfully treated with this medication, but the young man still needed surgeries to remove the lesions that did not respond. This story is an uncommon one, but it does highlight one of the potential health hazards of artificial tanning.

In my opinion, no one should use a tanning booth. Anyone who has a personal history of melanoma or other skin cancers *must not* use a tanning booth. If you have had any form of skin cancer, you should also tell your children and siblings to avoid tanning booths.

VI. Who Else in My Family Is at Risk for Developing Melanoma?

Most melanoma survivors are concerned about whether they are at risk for developing additional melanomas and whether their immediate relatives, especially their children, may develop melanoma at some point. The answers to these questions lie in understanding various risk factors. We know that individuals with certain genetic backgrounds, patterns of environmental exposure, and family histories are at higher risk. For those individuals, extra caution is needed to try to prevent melanoma.

What Are Your Skin Color and Hair Color?

Hair color, eye color, and skin color are determined by the genes we inherit from our parents. Some characteristics or appearances (called phenotypes) are more susceptible to developing melanoma than others. In general, people with blond or red hair, a fair complexion, and/or numerous freckles have a higher lifetime risk of developing melanoma than do individuals with a darker phenotype (darker skin, hair, and eyes). Individuals with a lighter phenotype tend to sunburn easily and do not tan. To categorize phenotypic differences, dermatologists have defined six skin types (called the Fitzpatrick scale of skin types), ranging from light to dark (table 3.3). Although people with any skin type can develop melanoma, individuals with skin types I, II, and III are at higher risk than people with the other skin types.

What Are Your Age and Sex?

Aside from the color of your hair, eyes, and skin, the factors of age and sex also play a role. Studies have shown that men tend to have a higher risk of developing skin cancer than women do. The higher incidence rate of melanoma seen in men can be attributed to the fact that men often do not protect themselves from UV exposure. Traditionally, men work outdoors more commonly than women and therefore have more cumulative sun exposure. In addition, some men do not like to use sunscreen.

People over 60 years old appear to have a higher risk. The higher incidence of melanoma seen in elderly people

Table 3.3. Fitzpatrick Skin Types

Skin type	Sunburning	Tanning	Other characteristics
I	Always burns	Never tans	Pale white skin, red or blond hair, blue or hazel eyes
II	Burns easily	Tans poorly	Fair skin
III	Burns	Tans after initial burn	Darker white skin
IV	Burns minimally	Tans easily	Light brown skin
V	Rarely burns	Tans darkly and easily	Brown skin
VI	Never burns	Tans quickly	Dark brown or dark skin

should not be a surprise. As we age, we accumulate DNA damage in our cells, resulting in a higher incidence of cancers of all types.

How Much Sun Exposure Have You Had?

Individuals with a history of intense and intermittent UV exposure have a higher-than-average lifetime risk of developing melanoma. UV exposure can come from the sun or from artificial sources such as tanning booths. UV radiation consists of short UV waves (UVB) and long UV waves (UVA). Both types of ultraviolet radiation can produce cellular and tissue damage. UVB causes direct damage to the DNA in skin cells, and UVA interacts with organelles (structures) in the tissue and generates oxygen radicals, which indirectly damage DNA. Individuals with a history of blistering or multiple sunburns, especially at an early age, have significantly higher risk for developing melanoma in adulthood.

Do You Have a Personal or Family History of Atypical Moles and Melanoma?

Individuals with a personal history or family history of melanoma are at higher risk for developing melanoma. In addition, individuals with many atypical (dysplastic) moles (nevi) have a higher risk. Table 3.4 presents the estimated increase in risk from the various melanoma risk factors. Some of the statistics are shocking. For example, compared to the risk for the general public, the risk of developing melanomas for individuals with many moles (more than 50) is 7 to 54 times higher. Individuals with

Table 3.4. Risk Factors for Developing Melanoma

Risk factors	Estimated relative risk*
Atypical nevi, prior melanoma, and familial melanoma	500
Large number of atypical nevi, familial melanoma, and no prior melanoma	148
Atypical nevi, no prior melanoma or familial melanoma	7–27
Many nevi (>50)	7–54
Giant congenital melanocytic nevi	101
Personal history of melanoma	9
History of melanoma in first-degree blood relatives	8
Immunosuppression	2–8
Red or blond hair and blue eyes	1–6

*Estimated relative risk means the number of times more likely a person with the characteristic(s) is to develop melanoma than is the average person.

some atypical moles but no personal or family history of melanomas are 7 to 27 times more likely to develop melanoma than people in the general population.

The most stunning statistic is the increase in risk for persons with a combination of atypical moles, prior personal history of melanoma, *and* a family history of melanoma. These individuals' likelihood of developing another melanoma is 500 times higher than that of the general public. That is why individuals with many moles, atypical moles, a prior personal history of melanoma, and a family history of melanoma should have frequent follow-up.

A full-body skin exam at least once a year is needed. Also, because a family history of melanoma is a risk factor, if you have melanoma, please tell your immediate blood relatives (e.g., children, siblings, and parents) that they should have at least a baseline skin examination. By telling them, you may save the life of someone you love.

Have You Had Any Non-melanoma Skin Cancer?

Individuals with actinic keratoses (a type of pre–skin cancer) or non-melanoma skin cancers (e.g., basal cell and squamous cell cancers) are at a higher risk for developing melanoma. All of these skin cancers are associated with increased UV exposure from the sun or artificial light sources. A history of non-melanoma skin cancer can be viewed as a surrogate marker, indicating chronic UV exposure and an increased risk for melanoma.

Do You Have Large Moles That Were Present at Birth?

Individuals with "giant" congenital moles have a higher risk of developing melanoma than the general public (*congenital* means "at birth"). Giant congenital moles are defined as moles that are larger than 20 cm in diameter in adulthood (they grow as the body grows). Although melanomas can develop in small- or medium-sized congenital moles, the occurrence of melanoma in them is much lower. An individual who was born with a large congenital mole generally should be monitored closely by health care providers for signs of melanoma.

Are You Immune Suppressed?

The immune system plays an important role in detecting and destroying melanoma. Immunotherapy leverages the body's innate immune system to destroy melanoma cells, so people with a suppressed immune system have a higher risk for developing melanoma. This includes individuals who are transplant recipients of solid organs (e.g., kidney, heart, or liver) or hematopoiesis (bone marrow). Transplant patients are required to take immune suppression drugs to prevent organ rejection. Other immune-suppressed individuals include patients with HIV infections.

Do You Have Any Genetic Predisposition?

Our genetic makeup plays a major role in determine the risk of developing melanoma. Before I get into some specific genes, I need to explain a few terms, namely, the difference between *somatic* and *germline* mutations. In general, germline mutations are passed down from your parents, as these mutations occur in the DNA of egg or sperm cells. These mutations affect all the cells in your body and can be passed on to your children. In contrast, somatic mutations occur in non-reproductive cells in the body. These cells make up the tissue and organs in the body but not the eggs or sperms that form the zygote (the first cell formed by the union of an egg and sperm). These mutations occur later in life, and we acquire them sporadically as we age. These mutations are not passed on to our offspring.

With that in mind, let me explain another pair of terms, namely, the difference between an *oncogene* and *tumor suppressor gene.* An oncogene is a gene that activates the growth and division of cells, and a tumor suppressor gene functions to slow the growth and division of cells. Mutation in either a tumor suppressor gene or an oncogene can lead to uncontrolled growth and proliferation of cells. To make an analogy to driving once again, having an oncogene mutation is like pushing the gas pedal to the floor, causing the car to speed down the highway. A mutation in the tumor suppressor gene is like having brakes that do not work, and the car cannot be stopped.

Let me now describe some important genes that contribute to the development of melanoma.

The first one is the *MC1R* gene (melanocortin 1 receptor). *MC1R* affects the production of melanin, the pigment that gives color to the skin, hair, and eyes. The *MC1R* gene has many natural variations. Some of these variations lead to the production of pheomelanin, which is seen in people with red hair, fair skin, and freckles. Pheomelanin is not as effective as eumelanin, a type of melanin seen in dark-skinned individuals, at protecting the body from UV radiation. In addition, upon UV exposure, pheomelanin becomes oxidative and releases free radicals that damage cells' organelles and the DNA in the genes. People with red hair variants of the *MC1R* gene have a higher risk of developing melanoma. They should protect themselves from UV exposure. For more information on *MC1R*, different types of melanin, and vitamin D, please see my interview with **Dr. David Fisher** (https://www .beatingmelanoma.com/david-fisher), a world-renowned dermatologist and physician scientist who studies the genetics of melanin.

1. Scan the code
2. Find the expert
3. Watch the interview

The second gene is *CDKN2A* (cyclin-dependent kinase inhibitor 2A). This is a tumor suppressor gene that helps to regulate cell growth and division. It subdues the activity of cyclin-dependent kinases and retinoblastoma protein, both of which function in controlling cell division. Mutations in this gene can be inherited (germline mutation), or they can be acquired later in life (somatic mutation). In both cases, mutations in this gene can increase the risk of melanoma and other cancers such as pancreatic and lung cancer.

The third gene is *PTEN* (phosphatase and tensin homolog), another tumor suppressor gene that helps to regulate cell growth and division. This gene mutation can occur in an inherited or acquired fashion. These mutations are present in a notable percentage of melanoma cases, especially in melanoma at an advanced stage. In addition, mutations in this gene are also found in prostate, breast, and endometrial cancers.

The fourth gene is *BAP1* (BRCA1-associated protein 1), another tumor suppressor gene that is located on chromosome 3p21.3. The BAP1 protein produced by the gene is involved in DNA repair, cell growth, and cell death. Mutations in the *BAP1* gene can increase the risk of developing melanoma of the skin. In addition, *BAP1* mutations are also found in uveal (eye) melanoma and mesothelioma.

The fifth gene is *BRCA1* (breast cancer 1, early onset), another tumor suppressor gene that is located on chromosome 17q21. The BRCA1 protein functions in DNA repair and cell cycle regulation. A mutation of this gene is most associated with the risk of breast and ovarian cancer, but it can also increase the risk of melanoma.

There are several other genes associated with the risk of developing melanoma. One thing to understand, though, is that having a mutation in any one of the genes described above does not automatically mean you will develop melanoma. Other health, environmental, and social factors also matter. For example, if you have a *CDKN2A* mutation and have extensive UV exposure, then your risk for developing melanoma will increase. In contrast, an individual with the same mutation who takes proper sun precautions will have a lower risk.

Before ending this section, I wish to touch on genetic counseling. Many patients with a history of melanoma ask whether they should have a genetic test to determine if they have any genes that predispose them and their family members to higher risk. In general, physicians become more alert when an individual has many melanomas (three or more), especially if they are relatively young. In addition, physicians become concerned when a patient has a family history of melanoma and other types of cancer (e.g., pancreatic or lung). Genetic counselors are the best-trained medical specialists to explore the need for genetic testing. For more details on genetic testing and genes related to melanoma, please see my interview with **Dr. Sancy Leachman** (https://www.beatingmelanoma.com/sancy-leachman), a melanoma expert and physician scientist, and with **Jeanne Homer** (https://www.beatingmelanoma.com/jeane -homer), a genetic counselor and the supervisor of Hoag's Hereditary Cancer Program.

1. Scan the code
2. Find the expert
3. Watch the interview

VII. Technological Innovations

Artificial Intelligence

Applications of artificial intelligence (AI) are becoming more prevalent in many industries, including in medicine. Nearly all of us have experienced the impact of AI in some aspects of our daily lives. Virtual assistants, such as Apple's Siri and Amazon's Alexa, can perform routine tasks ranging from answering simple questions to fulfilling our shopping requests. Tesla and other automakers are working to perfect autonomous vehicles. Smartphones can recognize your speech and transcribe your voice messages as texts or emails. ChatGPT can tell jokes and write romantic poems.

The use of AI or machine vision to detect melanoma and other skin cancer is not a new phenomenon. Nearly 20 years ago, I worked with a group of scientists and dermatologists in developing the first device approved by the FDA to detect melanoma. Unfortunately, the device failed to transfer from the research setting to the clinic.

Today, there are many companies and researchers around the world working collaboratively or independently to develop AI algorithms for distinguishing skin cancers from benign lesions. In most cases, the AI algorithms are trained on large data sets of clinical or dermoscopic images of skin lesions. The algorithms are then tested on a different data set of images to gauge their accuracy of detection. Beginning in 2019, researchers have published results showing that some AI algorithms performed better than dermatologists, even experts on melanoma, in detecting melanomas.

Advancements of AI in the detection of skin cancer offer a number of clinical benefits. First, AI can empower more health care providers to screen patients for melanoma, thereby catching it an early stage. Dermatologists are the specialists most skilled at detecting melanomas, but there is a shortage of dermatologists. A patient with a suspicious lesion may have to wait weeks or months before seeing a dermatologist. Second, AI can potentially enhance diagnostic accuracy, thereby improving the benign-to-malignant biopsy ratio. Put in simple terms, patients examined with the help of AI may not be subject to as many unnecessary biopsies. Diagnosing melanoma early while avoiding unnecessary biopsies has always been a goal for me and other melanoma experts. Lastly, empowered by AI, patients could perform more thorough self-exams and thus feel more confident in detecting skin cancer.

Despite tremendous progress, AI in its current state has a number of significant limitations. First, it is prone to data bias. Algorithms are only as good as the data they are trained on. If the data set used to train an AI model is not representative of the population it will be used on, the model may not perform well. For example, algorithms trained on lesion sets taken largely from Caucasian patients will not have a high accuracy rate in detecting melanomas in patients who are Asian, African American, or Hispanic.

The second limitation is inter-observer variability. Melanoma diagnosis is a complex task that relies on the interpretation of different clinical and dermoscopic features. There is a high degree of inter-observer variability in assessments made by dermatologists, and AI models may not be able to perform with any more consistency. Third, there is a lack of generalizability. That is, an AI model that performs well in one study may not perform as well in another study with a different test set of lesions. The fourth limitation is known as the "black box" phenomenon, where clinicians lack insight into how an algorithm has arrived at its diagnosis. That is, we do not understand what aspect of a lesion the AI is "looking" at or concerned about. Hence, it is hard to trust its decisions. Fifth is the difficult question of what to do when an AI's diagnosis differs from that of a human. This presents an ethical and legal conundrum.

So, what is the bottom line for the potential of AI in melanoma detection? We are at an inflection point. In the next few years, there is a high probability that some AI algorithms will be approved by the FDA and then deployed in clinical settings. My prediction is that AI will definitely help to detect melanoma early.

If you have more interest in this topic, please watch my interviews with **Dr. Allan Halpern** (https://www .beatingmelanoma.com/allan-c-halpern) and

Dr. Justin Ko (https://www .beatingmelanoma.com /justin-ko).

1. Scan the code
2. Find the expert
3. Watch the interview

Gene Expression Profiling

I have discussed in this chapter the interplay of genes and environmental factors in the risk of developing melanoma. In the previous chapter, I described targeted therapy, specifically BRAF and MEK inhibitors used to treat metastatic melanomas with a BRAF mutation. Here, in the last section, I want to profile four companies that have deployed new technologies to sample DNA and RNA from the skin or from biopsied specimens for diagnostic, prognostic, and therapeutic purposes.

DermTech Inc.

DermTech is a US company that has developed a noninvasive diagnostic test called a pigmented lesion assay. The assay uses adhesive tape to collect genetic information from lesions on the skin. It relies on the analysis of two RNA markers and one DNA marker. Based on the findings from these markers, the assay helps to predict whether a lesion is benign or malignant. If the assay predicts the lesion is benign, no skin biopsy is needed and the lesion can be monitored. If the assay predicts the lesion is malignant, the patient needs to have a biopsy to confirm the diagnosis of melanoma. In many cases, the biopsy and pathologic exam will show that the suspicious lesion is benign, despite the assay suggesting it could be malignant. The test has a high sensitivity (above 90 percent) and a specificity around 60 percent, which means that the assay is not always correct. The pigmented lesion assay is approved by the Food and Drug Administration and by the Conformité Européenne to distinguish melanoma from other benign pigmented skin lesions, such as atypical moles.

One area where this technology is very helpful is in assessing lesions on the face or other cosmetically sensitive areas in young or middle-aged people who do not want to have scars. Because the assay potentially reduces the need for a biopsy, it is an attractive alternative in these cases.

For more detailed information on DermTech technology, please watch my interview with **Dr. Laura Ferris** (https://www.beatingmelanoma.com/laura-ferris), a melanoma expert, dermatologist, and physician scientist who has conducted clinical trials on this technology.

1. Scan the code
2. Find the expert
3. Watch the interview

Castle Biosciences Inc.

Castle Biosciences is a US company that has developed a diagnostic test called DecisionDx-Melanoma, which uses gene expression profiling to classify patients with melanoma into low-risk, intermediate-risk, and high-risk groups. Unlike DermTech's assay, which samples the lesion on the skin, the Castle Biosciences test analyzes 31 genes in a melanoma biopsy sample. The process uses a proprietary algorithm to classify the melanoma samples into the three tiers of risk profiles. In addition, the company has developed another test called DecisionDX-UM, which is used to classify patients with uveal melanoma into different risk profiles.

These assays seem to show a potential to predict overall survival of patients with melanoma. However, it is not clear at this point how much more information these assays are providing in addition to the predictive data from the AJCC staging system based on tumor thickness, ulceration, and lymph node status. The assays are not foolproof.

For more detailed information regarding gene expression profiling and Castle Biosciences, please watch my interview with colleague **Dr. Douglas Grossman** (https://www.beatingmelanoma.com/douglas-grossman), a melanoma expert and physician scientist who has thoroughly studied this topic.

1. Scan the code
2. Find the expert
3. Watch the interview

SkylineDx Inc.

SkylineDX is a company in the Netherlands that has developed a diagnostic test called the Merlin Assay, which assesses the genetic profile of a melanoma biopsy sample. As mentioned in the last chapter, sentinel lymph node biopsy (SLNB) is a surgical procedure required to determine if a melanoma has spread to the lymph nodes. Remember that not all patients who meet the criteria for the procedure (e.g., a Breslow thickness of > 1 mm) will have a positive sentinel lymph node. Some statistics show that only 20 percent patients who undergo SLNB will test positive for disease. The Merlin Assay is designed to predict which patients may need an SLNB and which patients may not, based on gene expression profiling of the biopsied melanoma.

Caris Life Sciences Inc.

Caris Life Sciences is a US company that uses assays to profile DNA, RNA, and molecules with the goal of finding actionable therapeutic targets for cancer treatment. Unlike technologies relying on gene expression profiling, Caris uses next-generation sequence technology to analyze the genetic information of melanoma biopsy samples. Caris Molecular Intelligence technology analyzes over hundreds of genes, looking for specific gene mutations that can be targeted for treatment with existing FDA-approved drugs or drugs available in clinical trials.

For example, consider a patient with stage IV melanoma who is not responding to immunotherapy and who has developed new metastatic melanoma lesions on the skin and liver while undergoing Keytruda treatment. A biopsy of the new skin melanoma could be submitted for evaluation by Caris's technology. This technology can perhaps better characterize the mutation profiles of the melanoma, thus providing important information to suggest a suitable clinical trial or existing drug for the patient.

Gene expression profiling used to improve diagnosis, predict survival, and select therapeutic modalities will likely be important for the management of patients with melanoma and other types of cancers. At this time, however, there are still many limitations to these assays. In fact, the Melanoma Committee of the National Comprehensive Cancer Network and the American Academy of Dermatology have not endorsed any of these gene expression profiling tests as part of routine workup for patients with melanoma. Foreseeably in the future, though, new or improved assays will become part of standard care for patients with melanoma.

4. Networking

Finding and Sharing Information

We are nearing the end of this book. I hope that the information I presented in chapters 2 and 3 will help you navigate the "mad rush" phase of the melanoma journey. The five-step plan of chapter 2 is designed to reduce your anxiety and empower you as you interact with the medical professionals who will get you through this journey. Furthermore, I hope you have found answers to many of the common questions raised by melanoma survivors and their family members as they go through the "marathon" phase of the journey, the subject of chapter 3.

I am sure, though, that you will have some additional questions that I have not addressed in this book. Where else might you turn to find answers to these other questions? And where can you find support on your journey to recovery, both physically and emotionally?

Stay in Touch

By now, you should have already watched some of the in-depth interviews with experts that are available on BeatingMelanoma.com and the Beating Melanoma channel on YouTube. I am very grateful to all these melanoma experts who shared their insights. Their decades of research and clinical experience are a treasure trove of information.

I plan to interview more international experts and post additional videos about medical breakthroughs for the prevention, diagnosis, and treatment of melanoma. So, sign up for our newsletter at BeatingMelanoma.com and subscribe to the YouTube channel to get the latest updates.

Finally, if you have questions or suggestions, please submit them at BeatingMelanoma.com. Your feedback will help my colleagues and me provide better information for patients with melanoma.

Patient Support Communities

Gathering information is helpful. But many patients and melanoma survivors find that joining patient support communities is also valuable. You can find support groups either online or in your local community. In addition to learning about the firsthand experiences of others who are on the same journey, you will gain a sense of belonging. You are not alone. Fellow patients and survivors can provide the hope and inspiration that will help you cope with the physical and emotional effects of melanoma.

Sharing Your Stories

After beating melanoma, you will have made a difficult journey. You will remember the roller coaster of emotions and thoughts that you experienced in the "mad rush" phase. You will have knowledge and personal experience that can help other individuals with newly diagnosed melanoma. Although physicians are responsible for patient care, you can help too. By sharing your experience and offering advice, you can assist others in their moment of need. You are not just another patient; you are a melanoma survivor! The process of sharing your stories and experience can also be cathartic. Some of my patients have found a way to release their anxieties and fears by sharing their stories in support groups.

Giving Back

It is not uncommon for melanoma survivors to want to give back and help others. There are nonprofit organizations in this country that were launched to fight melanomas and other skin cancers. In addition to donating money to help these nonprofits, you can also support them with your time, expertise, connections, and skills. Any and all of these contributions will be appreciated. For example, one of my patients is a marketing director for a large wine distribution company in New Jersey. He hosts an annual wine tasting event and donates the proceeds to the Melanoma Foundation. One teenage patient created cartoon illustrations for a nonprofit company that uses the pictures to teach children about the importance of protecting themselves from excessive sun exposure.

Below are listed some of the medical associations, nonprofit organizations, and patient support groups that provide valuable information and resources for patients with melanoma. There are many more groups you can find online if you are interested in supporting your local organizations.

For more information on this topic, please watch my interviews with **Dan Latore** (https://www .beatingmelanoma.com/dan-latore), who is the executive director of the The Skin Cancer Foundation; **Dr. Deborah Sarnoff** (https://www.beatingmelanoma.com/deborah-s -sarnoff), who is the president of The Skin Cancer Foundation; and **Kyleigh LiPira** (https://www.beatingmelanoma .com/kyleigh-lipira), who is the CEO of the Melanoma Research Foundation. In addition to describing how you can give back, all three experts explain some valuable resources offered by these two foundations.

1. Scan the code
2. Find the expert
3. Watch the interview

Recommended Organizations and Their Websites

The Skin Cancer Foundation, https://www.skincancer.org/
Melanoma Research Foundation, https://melanoma.org/
American Academy of Dermatology, https://www.aad.org/
American Melanoma Foundation, https:// melanomafoundation.org/
American Cancer Society, https://www.cancer.org/
Melanoma International Foundation, https:// nationalmelanoma.org/
National Cancer Institute, https://www.nih.gov/about-nih /what-we-do/nih-almanac/national-cancer-institute-nci
Shade Foundation, http://shadefoundation.org/
Cancer Support Community, https://www .cancersupportcommunity.org/
AIM at Melanoma Foundation, https://www.aimatmelanoma .org/

5. Beating Melanoma Checklist

Chapter 2 provided a five-step plan for navigating the "mad rush" phase, and chapter 3 addressed many questions raised by melanoma survivors journeying through the "marathon" phase. This short chapter brings the information from chapters 2 and 3 together in an at-a-glance checklist. Even without the stress of a melanoma diagnosis, it is easy to forget or lose track of tasks when you have so many things to do. This checklist will, I hope, make it easier for you to work your way through the important steps in melanoma treatment and prevention.

1. "Mad Rush" Phase

☐ Obtain a physical copy of your pathology report.

☐ Read and understand the report.

    ☐ Where is my melanoma located?

    ☐ Is it in situ or invasive?

    ☐ What is the Breslow thickness?

    ☐ Is ulceration or mitosis present?

☐ Assess the reliability of the report. Do you and your physicians feel confident about the diagnosis?

☐ Determine the stage of melanoma by asking your doctor or by understanding the AJCC staging system. What is your stage?

    ☐ Stage 0 (i.e., melanoma in situ or lentigo maligna)

    ☐ Stage I

    ☐ Stage II

    ☐ Stage III (e.g., melanoma found in a clinically palpable lymph node or positive lymph node biopsy)

    ☐ Stage IV (e.g., melanoma has spread to other organs, such as liver, lung, or brain)

☐ Understand the treatment options. Discuss all the options with your doctors.

☐ Understand the survival outcomes. Discuss your prognosis with your doctors.

☐ Find melanoma experts in the area where you live.

2. "Marathon" Phase

☐ Are you seeing a dermatologist for a skin exam at least once a year?

- ☐ Is your doctor using a dermatoscope during the exam?
- ☐ Does your doctor look over your whole body?
- ☐ Are you routinely seeing an oncologist or a surgeon, if needed?
- ☐ How frequently are you visiting these doctors for follow-ups? Ask your doctor what he or she recommends for follow-up frequency, and then keep to that schedule.
- ☐ Determine your risk factors for developing additional melanomas.
- ☐ Do you have many (e.g., >50) atypical nevi?
  - ☐ If so, do you need total-body photography for a baseline documentation to track these moles?
- ☐ Are you doing monthly skin self-exams?
  - ☐ Do you have any lesions with the ABCDE features, "ugly duckling" sign, or symptoms of pain, itching, or bleeding?
- ☐ Are you preventing excessive UV exposure?
  - ☐ Do you wear protective clothing and a hat?
  - ☐ Do you seek shade to protect yourself?
  - ☐ Do you use sunscreen?
- ☐ Do you have a family or personal history of melanoma that indicates a need for genetic counseling?

3. Staying in Touch

- ☐ Sign up at BeatingMelanoma.com or subscribe to the Beating Melanoma channel on YouTube to receive updates.

Appendix A
Basal Cell Cancer

Every year, more than three million new cases of skin cancer are diagnosed in the United States. The most common type of skin cancer is basal cell cancer, which accounts for 80 percent of all diagnosed skin cancers. Basel cell cancers can grow and destroy surrounding tissue, especially if they are left untreated for a long time. Fortunately, basal cell cancer rarely spreads to other parts of the body.

Basal cell cancer, like other skin cancer, is caused mainly by excessive exposure to ultraviolet radiation. People with fair skin or who sunburn easily are at greatest risk for developing this cancer. Other potential risks for developing this cancer are a history of X-ray radiation, arsenic exposure, a major thermal burn, or a chronic wound that does not heal.

Most basal cell cancers are found on sun-exposed sites, such as the head, forehead, eyelids, nose, ears, neck, or back. There are many variants of basal cell cancer, with a wide range of presentations ("presentation" is doctor-talk for how they look and act).

One common type of basal cell cancer is the *nodular type*. It presents as a small pink or red nodule with a translucent appearance. Upon close inspection, small blood vessels may be visible. As the nodule grows, the center may become ulcerated.

Another common variant is the *superficial type.* Typically, it is a flat lesion that is pink or red in color. A small amount of scale may be seen on it.

Another type of basal cell cancer is the *morpheaform type.* Typically, this type has a raised texture and is an ivory color. Blood vessels may be seen in it.

Some basal cell cancers have dark pigmentation, or colors. Those are the *pigmented type.* Very often this variant can look like melanoma.

Treatment for basal cell cancer includes the following:

Mohs surgery
radiation
topical medication such as imiquimod
    cryotherapy
electrodessication and curettage
standard excision
photodynamic therapy

For more information about these treatments, talk with your doctor. Many of the organizations listed in chapter 4 can provide additional information about basal cell cancers and their treatment.

Examples of basal cell cancers are shown on Beating-Melanoma.com in color illustrations. Note, though, that basal cell cancers may have appearances other than those illustrated.

Appendix B
Squamous Cell Cancer

Of the more than three million new cases of skin cancer diagnosed in the United States each year, about 15 percent are squamous cell cancers, the second most common type of skin cancer. For most squamous cell cancers, the treatment is relatively straightforward, and the cure rate is excellent. There is a subset of squamous cell cancers, however, that are rather aggressive. They can cause extensive local tissue destruction and may recur after treatment. Some of these squamous cell cancers have the potential to spread to distant parts of the body and even lead to death.

As with other types of skin cancer, the cause of squamous cell cancer can be attributed to both environmental exposure and genetic predisposition. People with fair skin who sunburn easily are at greatest risk for developing this cancer. Ultraviolet radiation from the sun or other sources is the major culprit causing this skin cancer. More than 80 percent of all squamous cell cancers are found on sun-exposed surfaces such as the head, neck, and upper extremities. People who have received a transplanted organ are at an extremely high risk for developing this type of skin cancer because of the immunosuppressive drugs they must take. Other environmental exposure factors include soot, pitch and tar, shale oil, and arsenic.

The presentation of squamous cell cancer varies considerably ("presentation" means how these cancers look and act). In general, most squamous cell cancers develop on sun-damaged skin. The majority of squamous cell cancer patients have actinic keratosis, a type of precancerous spot that is red in color, has scales, and is rough to the touch. Most early squamous cell cancers have a rough scale. As the tumors grow, they enlarge into a nodule with or without ulceration. Large tumors can cause pain, can ulcerate, and can weep blood or other fluid.

Treatments for squamous cell cancer include the following:

Mohs surgery
radiation
topical medication such as imiquimod and
    5-fluorouracil
cryotherapy
electrodessication and curettage
standard excision photodynamic therapy

For more information about these treatments, talk with your doctor. Many of the organizations listed in chapter 4 can provide additional information about squamous cell cancer and its treatment.

Examples of squamous cell cancers are shown on BeatingMelanoma.com in color illustrations. Note, though, that squamous cell cancers may have appearances other than those illustrated.

Glossary

ABCDE. An abbreviation used to help the public and health care providers identify and remember clinical features of melanoma (*see* table 3.1).

actinic keratosis. A type of precancerous skin spot that is red in color, has scales, and is rough to the touch.

adjuvant therapy. Secondary treatment delivered to enhance the effectiveness of the primary treatment and help prevent recurrence of disease.

atypical nevi. Moles that resemble melanoma in appearance. Another name for these moles is dysplastic nevi.

basal cell carcinoma. The most common type of skin cancer.

benign. Normal. Not cancerous.

biopsy. Cutting away a small piece of skin tissue for diagnosis by microscopic examination.

blood count. The number of red cells, white cells, and platelets in a blood sample.

board certified. Physicians who have completed a requirement specified by their specialty board.

Breslow thickness. Measurement of the depth of penetration by tumor cells, taken from the top of the epidermis (outermost layer of the skin) to the deepest melanoma cells in the skin tissue.

cancer. A class of illnesses characterized by a proliferation of cells that invade and destroy normal surrounding tissue and have the potential to spread throughout the body.

CBC. Complete blood count. Measures the number of white blood cells, red blood cells, and platelets.

cell. The basic unit of a living organism.

centimeter (cm). A hundredth of a meter; about four-tenths of an inch.

chemotherapy. Treatment with a class of drugs used to destroy cancer.

Clark's level. A way for pathologists to report the depth of melanoma invasion.

clinical trial. A medical study evaluating the efficacy of experimental treatments for cancer or other diseases.

confocal laser microscopy. An imaging method designed to examine the cellular structures within skin tissue in a noninvasive fashion.

congenital mole. A mole present at birth. The size of a congenital mole can vary from a few millimeters to larger than 20 centimeters in diameter.

cryotherapy. Treatment that freezes benign or malignant skin lesions with liquid nitrogen.

CT scan. Computed tomography scan. A series of X-ray views of the body from different angles. The images are combined and reconstructed by computer and reviewed by a radiologist. Sometimes called a CAT (computerized axial tomography) scan.

cure rate. The percentage of patients with a disease who have been cured, as determined by statistical studies.

curettage. A method of treating skin cancer by scraping away the tumor cells.

dermatologist. A physician who specializes in diagnosing and treating skin problems.

dermatoscope (or dermoscope). A handheld microscope-like device that allows physicians to see deeper layers of the skin than are visible to the naked eye and in a noninvasive fashion.

dermis. The lower layer of the skin found immediately below the epidermis (outermost) layer.

DNA (deoxyribonucleic acid). Nucleic acids containing the genetic information of living organisms.

dysplastic nevi. *See* **atypical nevi.**

electrodessication. A method of treating benign or malignant skin lesions using high-energy electrical currents or heat.

epidermis. The outermost or uppermost layer of the skin, located above the dermis layer.

excisional biopsy. A surgical procedure in which a piece of tumor or skin tissue is removed. The specimen is examined under a microscope for diagnosis.

Food and Drug Administration (FDA). A division of the federal government that regulates the safety and efficacy of drugs.

freckles. Light brown pigmentations found on the skin.

gene. A strand of DNA molecules needed by cells to produce proteins.

gene expression profiling. A method of measuring which genes, thousands in some instances, are being expressed in a cell at any given moment.

gene therapy. Treatment that targets gene mutations.

groin. The area of the body where the thighs meet the hip and abdomen.

high-risk melanoma. Aggressive or advanced-stage melanoma that has a high probability of coming back, or recurring.

immune system. The body's defensive mechanism for combating illness. It is an elaborate system composed of different types of immune cells that work together to seek, identify, and destroy viruses, bacteria, and cancer cells.

immunosuppression. A condition, caused by illness or certain therapies, in which the effectiveness of a person's immune system is reduced.

immunotherapy. A type of cancer treatment that boosts the body's immune system to destroy cancer.

in situ. Latin for "in place," in this case meaning "in the original place." Used in reference to a skin cancer that is restricted to the epidermis, the top layer of the skin.

intravenous (IV). Into a vein. Usually describes medicine being delivered through the bloodstream.

lentigo maligna. A type of melanoma in situ lesion.

lesion. Abnormal tissue found on or in the body. It can be either benign or malignant.

lymphedema. Swelling of the arm or leg due to an accumulation of excess lymphatic fluid. The condition commonly occurs in patients who have had surgical procedures to remove lymph vessels or lymph nodes.

lymph nodes. Small bean-shaped immunologic structures (*see also* **immune system**) connected to the lymphatic vessels, which are found throughout the body. They contain various immunologic cells (e.g., T and B cells) and can become enlarged or painful when the body is fighting illnesses ranging from infection to cancer.

malignant. Cancerous. Malignant tumors or cells can destroy nearby normal tissue and can spread to other parts of the body.

melanocyte. A specialized pigment-producing cell located in the bottom layer of the epidermis. Melanoma is derived from cancerous melanocytes.

melanoma. A type of skin cancer derived from cancerous melanocytes.

metastasis. The spread of cancer cells from one part of the body to another part of the body via the bloodstream or the lymphatic system.

metastatic melanoma. Melanoma that has spread from the original site to other parts of the body, such as bone, brain, liver, or other parts of the skin.

mitosis or **mitotic rate.** The multiplication of cells by division, whereby one cell splits into two cells. Mitotic rate is a measurement of the rate of cell division.

mole. A collection of melanocytes in the skin. A mole appears as a brown, black, or flesh-colored spot on the skin. Also called a nevus.

MRI. Magnetic resonance imaging. A medical imaging technique used to visualize internal structures of the body.

neurotropism. Presence of cancer cells in nerves.

nevus (plural, **nevi**). *See* **mole.**

nodule. A type of growth found in the body.

oncologist. A physician who specializes in treating cancer.

pathologist. A physician who specializes in diagnosing diseases by examining tissues and cells under a microscope.

PET scan. Positron emission tomography scan. A nuclear imaging technology capable of detecting areas of the body that contain malignant cells.

photodynamic therapy. A method of treating benign or malignant skin lesions using a combination of light and chemicals.

plastic surgeon. A surgeon who specializes in restoring function and normal appearance to parts of the body altered by disease, injury, or surgery (such as for the removal of cancerous lesions).

prognosis. A prediction of the probable outcome of a disease.

radiation oncologist. A physician who specializes in radiation treatment for cancer.

recurrence. The reappearance of a cancer or disease after a period of remission.

remission. Disappearance of a cancer or chronic illness.

resection. Surgical removal of tissue, such as a malignant tumor.

RNA. Ribonucleic acid is produced from DNA and is important in protein production.

sentinel lymph node. The first lymph node or nodes that malignant tumor cells reach when cancer spreads from its original site.

sentinel lymph node biopsy (SLNB). A surgical procedure to remove and examine the sentinel lymph node to determine if cancerous cells are present.

side effect. A secondary effect, sometimes harmful, of a drug or therapy that may occur in addition to the primary effect.

SPF. Sun protection factor. A standard for measuring the efficacy of sunscreen in protecting against (mainly) the UVB portion of solar radiation.

squamous cell carcinoma. A type of skin cancer.

sunscreen. A substance applied to the skin to block or reflect ultraviolet radiation from the sun.

survival rate. The percentage of patients with a particular disease who survived after treatment, as determined by statistical studies.

targeted therapy. A type of cancer treatment that targets a specific protein that drives the growth of cancer cells.

tumor. An abnormal growth of tissue. A tumor can be either benign (not cancerous) or malignant (cancerous).

ulceration. Open area on the skin or in tissue where there is breakdown of the normal structure.

ultrasound. An imaging procedure using sound waves to visualize soft tissue and body cavities.

ultraviolet (UV) radiation. A spectrum of invisible rays from the sun or a sun lamp. UV radiation can cause skin cancer and can accelerate aging. UVA rays have a longer wavelength than UVB rays.

vitamin D. A fat-soluble vitamin that helps strengthen bones and can be generated by the body from sun exposure or obtained from food sources or vitamin supplements.

Index

Page references in *italic* indicate a figure; page references in **bold** indicate a table.

About the Author

Steven Q. Wang, MD, a dermatologist and Mohs surgeon, currently serves as the director of the Dermatologic Oncology Program at the Hoag Family Cancer Institute in California. Prior to joining Hoag Memorial Hospital Presbyterian, Dr. Wang served as the director of Dermatologic Surgery and Dermatology at Memorial Sloan Kettering Cancer Center in New Jersey. He specializes in the prevention, diagnosis, and treatment of skin cancers, especially melanoma. In managing the care of high-risk skin cancer patients, he uses total-body photography, dermoscopy, and computerized digital imaging systems. He is also actively involved in clinical research, with a focus on photoprotection and noninvasive imaging technologies to diagnose skin cancer. He has authored more than 90 publications in peer-reviewed medical journals and textbooks. He is the author or editor of five books and has lectured extensively in the United States and around the world on the diagnosis, treatment, and prevention of melanoma and non-melanoma skin cancers.

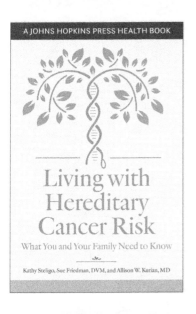
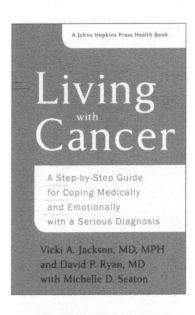
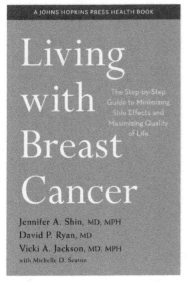
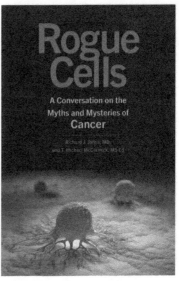